# COMMUNICATION SKILLS IN NURSING, HEALTH & SOCIAL CARE

Sara Miller McCune founded SAGE Publishing in 1965 to support the dissemination of usable knowledge and educate a global community. SAGE publishes more than 1000 journals and over 800 new books each year, spanning a wide range of subject areas. Our growing selection of library products includes archives, data, case studies and video. SAGE remains majority owned by our founder and after her lifetime will become owned by a charitable trust that secures the company's continued independence.

Los Angeles | London | New Delhi | Singapore | Washington DC | Melbourne

( BERNARD MOSS )

# COMMUNICATION SKILLS IN NURSING, HEALTH & SOCIAL CARE

## 5TH EDITION

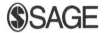

Los Angeles | London | New Delhi
Singapore | Washington DC | Melbourne

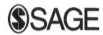

Los Angeles | London | New Delhi
Singapore | Washington DC | Melbourne

SAGE Publications Ltd
1 Oliver's Yard
55 City Road
London EC1Y 1SP

SAGE Publications Inc.
2455 Teller Road
Thousand Oaks, California 91320

SAGE Publications India Pvt Ltd
B 1/I 1 Mohan Cooperative Industrial Area
Mathura Road
New Delhi 110 044

SAGE Publications Asia-Pacific Pte Ltd
3 Church Street
#10-04 Samsung Hub
Singapore 049483

Editor: Kate Keers/Catriona McMullen
Assistant editor: Talulah Hall/Ruth Lilly
Production editor: Martin Fox
Copyeditor: Solveig Gardner Servian
Proofreader: Rebecca Storr
Marketing manager: Camille Richmond
Cover design: Wendy Scott
Typeset by: C&M Digitals (P) Ltd, Chennai, India
Printed in the UK

**Library of Congress Control Number: 2019949836**

**British Library Cataloguing in Publication data**

A catalogue record for this book is available from
the British Library

ISBN 978-1-5264-9015-5
ISBN 978-1-5264-9014-8 (pbk)

At SAGE we take sustainability seriously. Most of our products are printed in the UK using responsibly sourced
papers and boards. When we print overseas we ensure sustainable papers are used as measured by the PREPS
grading system. We undertake an annual audit to monitor our sustainability.

In memory of Bernard Moss
1944–2020

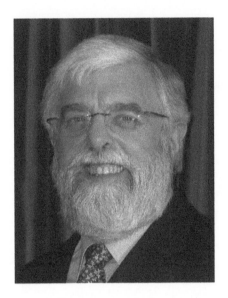

He will be deeply missed by his wife Sheila, his extended family and many
friends, all those who worked with him and who benefitted from his skills and
care as a minister of religion and educator.

This fifth edition owes so much to the wisdom and experience of valued colleagues, particularly Kate Bebe, Professor Liz Boath, Tracy Pestana and Kim Sargeant, together with the advice work team at Staffordshire University. Their contributions have enriched this edition and will deepen the learning that readers will achieve when engaging with the issues we raise.

As always, I thank my wife Sheila, without whose unfailing love and encouragement none of this would have happened.

This edition is dedicated to Penny, who has already enriched the lives of more people than she will probably ever realise.

# CONTENTS

# ABOUT THE AUTHOR

Bernard Moss was Emeritus Professor of Social Work Education and Spirituality at Staffordshire University. He was responsible for teaching communication skills to social work students for over a decade. His highly interactive and experiential approach to teaching gave students an opportunity to take responsibility for their own learning and development as trainee practitioners. His teaching excellence was recognised by the Higher Education Academy UK, who in 2004 awarded him a National Teaching Fellowship, in 2007 a Senior Fellowship, and in 2013 Principal Fellowship status.

He was part of the working group established by the Social Care Institute for Excellence to prepare a report on the literature on communication skills for social work, and also produced a DVD on the use of large-group role play in higher education. He was one of only three UK university teachers to be invited to contribute a chapter to the prestigious international publication *Inspiring Academics: Learning with the World's Great University Teachers*, published in 2011 by Open University Press.

He published widely on the theme of spirituality, for which he was awarded a PhD by Staffordshire University in 2011. His book on *Spirituality and Social Work* (Palgrave), co-authored with Professor Margaret Holloway in 2010, has been widely acclaimed.

In 2016, he co-authored with Dr Jan Sellers an international book on the use of labyrinths in higher education and the contribution that labyrinth walks can make to enrich the learning and teaching process for students and staff, as well as enhancing their general wellbeing (*Learning with the Labyrinth: Creating Reflective Space in Higher Education*, Palgrave Macmillan).

In 2019, he co-authored an article for the educational journal of the Royal College of General Practitioners on the role of simulated patients helping trainee GPs prepare for the Clinical Skills Assessment examination (*InnovAiT*, Vol. 12, Issue 1).

# ABOUT THE CONTRIBUTORS

## KATE BEBE

Kate Bebe is a qualified and registered social worker. As a Lecturer in Social Work at Staffordshire University she is mainly responsible for students' practical learning experiences. She has more than 32 years' experience in social care and social work across numerous adult service user areas within a Local Authority setting. She played an instrumental role in the implementation of the Single Assessment Process as part of the National Service Framework 2001.

Since 2003, initially alongside her Local Authority role, Kate has been involved in the BA and MA social work programmes at several universities across the North West and Midlands, teaching communication skills in students' first year of study and delivering other module-based learning in line with the curriculum.

During that time and up to the present day, Kate has been an independent off-site Practice Educator. She is dedicated to practice education and the promotion of placement experience alongside academic learning. She is particularly passionate about group supervision, group learning activities with the emphasis upon learning from others, and service user involvement in students' skill-based learning.

Her other interests include the promotion of end-of-life care choice and reducing age discrimination.

## LIZ BOATH

Liz Boath is Professor of Health and Wellbeing at Staffordshire University where she is a Teaching Excellence Fellow. She was awarded a National Teaching Fellowship by the Higher Education Academy in 2007 and later became a Senior Fellow in recognition of her teaching excellence and innovative contributions to Higher Education.

Liz has a background in psychology and is a Certified Advanced Emotional Freedom Techniques (EFT) Practitioner. She has made seminal contributions to EFT Research and has pioneered the use of EFT with University students to reduce exam stress and presentation anxiety. She is also a Clinical Hypnotherapist and a coach and mentor.

Liz has a PhD in Perinatal Mental Health and has over three decades' experience in health and social care education and research. She is the Research Lead for the

School of Health and Social Care at Staffordshire University and has a keen interest in ethics.

She has co-authored eight books, six book chapters and written over 60 peer reviewed publications and presented at over 90 national and international conferences.

## TRACY PESTANA

Tracy Pestana trained at Staffordshire University and is a qualified social worker with wide experience in a variety of Local Authority settings. This includes work in Child Safeguarding and Looked After Children, and Unaccompanied Asylum-Seeking Children. Her current role involves work with adults who reside in the prison system. She continues to work in child protection as a member of her local Emergency Duty Team.

Tracy is committed to the importance of clear, positive relationship building, both with service users and other professionals, as well as the communication skills that are pivotal for effective social work. She has received several commendations from service users and other professionals for the quality of her work and the social work values she embodies. Although realistic about what social workers can achieve, she emphasises the importance of good supervision and reflective practice as essential components of best practice.

Tracy's advice is: never be afraid to ask a question and never give up!

## KIM SARGEANT

Kim Sargeant is a nurse lecturer at Keele University where she is the Director of Education for the School of Primary, Community and Social Care, and the Deputy Director for Learning and Teaching for the School of Nursing and Midwifery.

Her background is as a Registered Nurse, Registered Midwife and a Registered Nurse Teacher. She has over 20 years' experience of teaching nurse education in both Further and Higher Education settings. As an experienced nurse lecturer she teaches at undergraduate, postgraduate, pre-registration and post-registration levels within the School of Nursing and Midwifery.

Her interests are in education, particularly in curriculum design, assessment and quality, with a special interest in Professional Nursing Standards. She has presented her work at several international conferences. Kim has also written and implemented a number of curricula developments and has made significant contributions in educating clinical and academic staff in the support and education of student nurses during their pre-registration studies.

Her doctoral research has explored the perceptions of newly qualified nurses and their preparation for the realities of working as a qualified nurse in contemporary practice.

# FOREWORD

## DR NEIL THOMPSON

I have long been fascinated by language in particular and communication in general. Throughout my professional career, I have been aware of how central communication is to the effectiveness or otherwise of our endeavours – and how drastically wrong things can turn out when people do not attach sufficient significance to communication, or fail to treat it with the respect it deserves.

This book, from a highly respected educator and author, with a wealth of experience and expertise in the 'people professions', is therefore one that I very much welcome. The author's extensive knowledge base – and skill in communicating it effectively – is amply evidenced in this important work. What comes across very clearly is that here is someone who not only has an excellent grasp of the subtleties of communication as an academic discipline, but also fully understands how the theoretical underpinnings manifest themselves in the complex world of professional practice. And, as if that were not enough in itself, he also 'practises what he teaches' (there is no preaching here!), in so far as he conveys in a highly effective way his important messages about communication skills in action.

There are many books to be found on the subject of communication that are not of direct use to professional practitioners. Some are highly abstract tomes that explore certain issues in fine detail and, while there may be some important indirect, longer-term lessons to be learned from such works, their immediate value to the busy practitioner or manager is limited. Other books on communication provide a 'cookbook', how-to type slant on the subject – often risking the dangers of oversimplification that can arise from such approaches. Communication is far too complex and important a topic to be left to such a simplistic approach. There are, then, relatively few books that provide a helpful blend of theory and practice, but this fine work is certainly one of them – and what an excellent one it is too.

The use of what might be called an enhanced dictionary format (enhanced, in the sense that it is not simply a set of basic definitions, but rather is enriched by commentary, learning exercises and so on) is particularly effective in providing both an overview of the territory and helpful guidance on linking theoretical understanding to the challenges of practice. This is no doubt what has made this a popular and successful book, and deservedly so.

High-quality professional practice is not possible without a high level of communicative effectiveness. This book will therefore be a significant contribution to developing the foundations of effective communication and thus paving the way for the high-quality practice the people we serve are entitled to.

I am delighted that this important book is now available in a further revised, updated and expanded edition. It builds on the strengths of the first four editions and offers a range of important new insights and therefore even more value. This is good news for students, practitioners and managers across health, social care and beyond, as there can be no substitute for effective communication. This excellent book has gone from strength to strength with each new edition. The fact that it has now reached its fifth edition shows clearly what an invaluable resource it is. I wish I had had this book available to me when I was a practitioner.

Sadly, shortly before this edition went to print, Bernard Moss passed away. He had been my friend and colleague for over 25 years, and what an excellent friend and colleague he was. As this book amply illustrates, Bernard had an outstanding grasp of what it means to be human, constantly interacting with other humans in meaningful ways. He was an inspiring teacher, much loved by students and colleagues alike. His kindness and generosity of spirit were just some of his highly endearing qualities. The world is much diminished by his loss and that makes this book even more of a learning resource to be treasured.

Dr Neil Thompson, independent writer and online tutor
(www.NeilThompson. info)

# FOREWORD

## BISHOP SARAH MULLALLY

Good communication is central to good care. Not only does it result in more accurate, safe, effective and efficient care, but it also promotes the wellbeing and satisfaction of those being cared for and the wellbeing of those caring.

To achieve this there is a need to understand those being cared for, demonstrating courtesy, kindness and sincerity. Good communication is not only based on the physical abilities of the carer, but also on education and experience. Whilst all of us have communication skills we can all benefit from developing them more intentionally. Our skills are further enhanced if we undertake this development with other people.

We are all parts of multi-disciplinary teams and diversity is critical to their effectiveness. Teamwork is a complex process in which different types of staff work together to share expertise, knowledge, and skills to impact on care, but the reality is, that working together from a variety of perspectives is sometimes difficult to achieve.

This book provides a tool for use by groups of health and social care professionals to enhance communication skills. It is a wonderful blend of theory and practice. Learning undertaken in multi-professional groups will further develop an ability to achieve objectives. In doing so I hope that care will be better focused around the individual and more effective and that professional satisfaction will be increased.

Bernard Moss was a highly respected educator and his vast experience is evident on every page. This book has made an important contribution to health and social care education for several years and his recent passing is a great loss to the field. I am confident that the distilled wisdom contained in this book will continue to aid professionals working in these areas for many generations to come.

The Rt Revd and Rt Hon Dame Sarah Mullally

Bishop of London and Former Chief Nursing Officer for England

# ACKNOWLEDGEMENTS

No book is ever written in a vacuum. My own development in communication skills is a rich tapestry of experience, beginning as a worker in a community therapy psychiatric hospital in the 1960s, training as a faith community leader, then as a relationship counsellor, and later as a family mediator and as a probation officer. For over a decade or so, I had the lead responsibility for teaching communication skills to social work students at Staffordshire University, involving members of the Service User and Carers Group who play a key role in working with students to practise and develop their basic communication skills. Under my leadership this group won a Community Care Excellence Award in 2009, and the prestigious award from the Social Work and Social Policy Subject Centre, Higher Education Academy UK in 2011 for their pioneering innovative work in delivering communication skills training. I owe a huge debt of gratitude to them for their enthusiastic commitment.

I have been privileged to work as a member of the simulated patient team at Keele University helping trainee doctors with their communication skills. With my colleagues in Moss Enterprises we have developed and delivered communication/customer care skills workshops for receptionists in GP practices, and with Neil Thompson have produced a training DVD on best practice in customer care. Within the West Midlands area we have contributed to the communication skills training of doctors at various stages in their professional development. For this work my wife and I were presented with a Quality Award in General Practice Training and Education by the Royal College of GPs in 2014. To everyone who has made such opportunities available to us we are most grateful.

My career has recently come full circle through a new ministry as Associate Minister in St Mary's Church Nantwich, the 'cathedral' of South Cheshire, with opportunities to share journeys with people, to listen to their life stories, and to offer hope and encouragement. I hope that other colleagues in faith community leadership will find much of this book helpful and encouraging in their important work.

For this fifth edition I am especially grateful to several colleagues for their professional expertise, experience and wisdom, whose contributions have enhanced this book. They include Professor Liz Boath, Kate Bebe both from Staffordshire University; Tracy Pestana an experienced social work practitioner and colleague; Kim Sargeant from Keele University whose national reputation in nursing education and practice has enabled this book to speak to nursing students. The team at SAGE have been unstinting in their encouragement to me throughout this project. They have made me feel that I have something useful to say, and it has been a privilege to work with them.

In the end, of course, the buck stops with me, and any grumbles belong in my in-tray alone.

# INTRODUCTION TO THE FIFTH EDITION

This fifth edition seeks to respond to some important feedback to the previous edition. Significantly, increasing numbers of nursing students have begun to use this book even though previous editions have not specifically addressed the communication skills needs of this profession. Most of the issues addressed in the book are already relevant to a wide range of people-workers, but this fifth edition brings an opportunity to develop a nursing focus to enrich the book's overall appeal.

Another feature has been the development of a wider set of activities to help students and practitioners engage more deeply and reflectively with key issues, not just as individuals but in a group learning context. Tutors across many disciplines are always looking for relevant interactive ways of enhancing student learning in small and large groups, and I am grateful to Kate Bebe of Staffordshire University for contributing the 'group exercises' to this new edition.

## PROFESSIONAL STANDARDS

The context and impact of professional standards remains central to all professional people-work by establishing professional expectations and boundaries within which we work with those committed to our care. With an ever-increasing readership of this book by nursing students it is important to introduce the new Code of Professional Practice as part of the Introduction. This will help nursing students feel more 'at home' when using the book; but equally important in days when interprofessional collaboration is essential, it will enable other professions to understand and learn from the hard work being undertaken in this field by other disciplines. I am grateful therefore to Kim Sargeant from Keele University for her contributions to the book and the following detailed exploration of the relevance of professional standards to everyday practice, specifically for nurses but more generally for all people-work. The British Association of Social Workers has continued to develop the Professional Capabilities Framework which enables social workers and social care workers to understand, and work to, a set of professional standards (Figure 1).

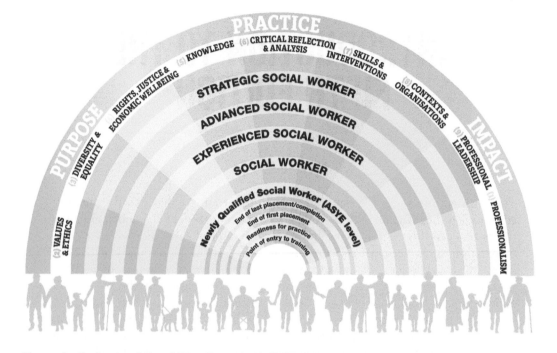

**Figure 1**   Professional Capabilities Framework (PCF) for social workers

*Source*: © British Association of Social Workers, 2018. Published with kind permission of BASW – www.basw.co.uk.

## PROFESSIONAL STANDARDS FOR NURSES

The Nursing and Midwifery Council (NMC), is the professional body that oversees and regulates nurses and midwives within the United Kingdom. As part of their role, they set the professional standards that must be achieved for entry to the professional register as a qualified nurse, midwife or nursing associate. They also produce the Code of Professional Conduct, known as 'the Code' (NMC, 2018a), which details the standards that all student and qualified nurses, midwives and nursing associates must abide by in order to protect the public and to promote high quality professional care from all nurses, midwives and nursing associates. To ensure that the education undertaken by nursing students is appropriate and relevant, the standards relating to that education are reviewed periodically and updated by the NMC.

In the rapidly changing healthcare landscape, it is important that student nurses are educated to meet the demands of contemporary nursing practice. In 2018 the NMC introduced new professional standards under the title 'Future Nurse: Standards of Proficiency for Registered Nurses'. These new standards aim to prepare the next generation of nurses for their professional role in modern-day nursing. Within these standards are the standards framework for nursing and midwifery education, the standards for student supervision and assessment, and the specific standards for the pre-registration nursing programme. These standards are significant as they guide and inform the development of the pre-registration nursing curriculum, and the support and assessment of students in both theory and clinical practice. The new Future Nurse Standards bring about a number of changes to the way that student nurses are supported to learn, and the focus of that learning.

## PROFICIENCIES

To enable the student to demonstrate that they have the knowledge, skills and attributes required of a qualified nurse, they must demonstrate achievement of a number of proficiencies. These reflect the expectations of the Newly Qualified Nurse on entry to the professional register. The current system of mentoring in clinical practice is shortly to be replaced by a model which encourages more of a coaching approach. Rather than being supported and assessed by a mentor, students will now be supported by a Practice Supervisor and assessed by a separate Practice Assessor for each part of their programme. Students will also have an Academic Assessor who will confirm the student's achievement of the programme proficiencies and who will work in partnership with the Practice Assessor. These changes will allow for greater flexibility in the learning opportunities available to student nurses, whilst ensuring that the professional standards set by the NMC are met.

## PLATFORMS

The new standards take a more holistic approach to the education of nursing students, with greater recognition of the generic qualities, skills and knowledge that all nurses must have, regardless of their field of nursing (adult, child, learning disabilities, mental health).

Therefore, the proficiencies have been grouped into sections known as 'Platforms'. The proficiencies within each Platform must be achieved by all new graduate nurses, with the addition of some advanced skills related to the specific needs of the different fields of nursing practice. Achievement of these proficiencies will then prepare the Newly Qualified Nurse for their career as a professional graduate nurse and for their ongoing knowledge and skills development.

The seven Platforms that house the new proficiencies are:

1   Being an accountable professional
2   Promoting health and preventing ill health
3   Assessing needs and planning care
4   Providing and evaluating care
5   Leading and managing nursing care and working in teams
6   Improving safety and quality of care
7   Coordinating care

Leadership and management are a key focus for the next generation of registered nurses with a greater expectation to manage and coordinate care from an early point in their career. The new role of the Nursing Associate will support the qualified nurse in their care and management of service users with increasingly complex care needs. Whilst the Nursing Associate will be a stand-alone role, regulated by the Nursing and Midwifery Council, the Newly Qualified Nurse will be expected to coordinate and manage the care delivered by the Nursing Associate.

## COMMUNICATION AND RELATIONSHIP MANAGEMENT

Within nursing, communication has always been a key and vital skill, to ensure that high quality individualised person-centred care is provided. Within the new Future Nurse Standards, the role of communication continues to have key emphasis, with Annex A focusing specifically on Communication and Relationship Management skills. In recognition of the importance of communication for nurses, and the diverse skills required for the provision of high-quality nursing care, these Communication and Relationship Management skills are broken down into four areas:

1   Underpinning communication skills for assessing, planning, providing and managing best practice, evidence-based nursing care
2   Evidence-based, best practice approaches to communication for supporting people of all ages, their families and carers in preventing ill health and in managing their care
3   Evidence-based, best practice communication skills and approaches for providing therapeutic interventions
4   Evidence-based, best practice communication skills and approaches for working with people in professional teams

The aim of this book therefore is to help nursing students, alongside other professionals, in their development of these Communication and Relationship Management skills.

## THE AIMS OF THE BOOK

This book is aimed at any of the helping professions for whom good communication skills are an essential part of their role. It was originally written for social worker students, not least because the author is deeply involved in social work education and has many years' experience in helping students develop their communication skills for this important work. But in these days of multi-disciplinary and interprofessional collaboration, it cannot be argued that there is a set of communication skills that is uniquely relevant to any one profession or discipline. Communication skills are essential skills, and it behoves anyone working with other people to take the responsibility for ensuring that these skills are developed to the highest level possible.

For this reason, the admittedly somewhat inelegant term 'people-worker' has been adopted throughout. If you are involved in any way at all, with an agency that sets out to help people and offer support, professionally or in a voluntary capacity, then this book is for you. Social workers, probation officers, doctors, nurses and paramedics, teachers, police officers, youth workers, advice workers, faith community leaders, and many others who work in a wide range of 'not-for-profit' helping agencies: these colleagues are the audience that this book seeks to address. Inevitably, there will be issues which have not been covered, or which some disciplines feel should have been given a different focus. No book can be everything to all its readers. Nevertheless, the issues covered here are widely relevant, and the activities included here can be used and applied by colleagues in a wide range of settings. The book is designed to stimulate and develop reflection about how to improve communication skills, and therefore also depends significantly upon the amount of energy and enthusiasm put into it by the reader to maximise its benefits.

## A DICTIONARY APPROACH

The design of the book deserves some comment. There are many excellent books already on the market dealing with communication skills for particular professional groups, many of them taking their readers into great depth and great detail. This book does not in any way seek to replace such volumes, or to suggest that they do not repay careful, prolonged and detailed study. They remain core texts for various disciplines. This dictionary approach, with its relevance to a variety of professional disciplines, has been adopted for the following reasons:

- It seeks to be more accessible, by drawing together the main themes for a specific topic into one discussion. In many of the other core texts on the market, the reader often has to consult the index and then several different pages in order to gain a full picture.
- It acts as both an introduction for a student and as a refresher to the busy practitioner. Key issues and themes are identified to provide a good grasp and overview of the particular topic, with encouragement to more in-depth study by suggesting further reading and deeper reflection.
- It seeks to be especially helpful to mentors, practice educators, supervisors and other experienced colleagues who have responsibility to help trainees and students develop their communication skills, and to develop their awareness. The activities offered throughout the book may be used, therefore, as group or individual discussion starters or in preparation for supervision. Its accessible, even conversational, style reflects a relationship between a tutor/supervisor/trainee and a worker or student. It seeks to talk with the reader about important themes in an encouraging and facilitative way so that they can develop their own style with confidence.

There are nevertheless some challenges to this approach. No book can ever be totally comprehensive, and inevitably there will be some readers who feel that the choice of topics has been incomplete. There is also the difficulty of avoiding unnecessary repetition. To help achieve this, some themes have been brought together into a more general discussion. The themes of resilience and a strengths perspective, for example, are discussed under the heading of Empowerment, and some of the core aspects of active listening have been explored under that heading rather than commanding several individual entries, in order to help achieve a coherent approach. The reader is signposted to these general discussions where necessary.

## INTRODUCING COMMUNICATION SKILLS

Implicit throughout this is a comprehensive understanding of what is meant by communication skills for people-work. There are, of course, some very specific skills and techniques, such as the use of open questions and genograms, which may be seen as the people-worker's equivalent of the carpenter's ability to make mortise and tenon joints accurately. These are skills that can be identified and practised as part of the worker's communication skills toolkit, and will help them to do a better job. But communication is a far more complex phenomenon than a set of discrete skills. It is something to do with the whole person, the context in which you work, and ultimately the societal values that serve as a backdrop for the work you undertake. For this reason, the entries in this book will be more than a set of definitions; they offer a far more wide-ranging and discursive approach, and will seek to track the 'ripples in the pond' that your interventions with people create. There will be some entries, therefore, which tackle a certain key theme in people-work and invite you to explore what communication skills will be important in order to deal successfully with this topic. One example of this is the entry on Breaking Bad News. This skill is beginning to feature strongly in the communication skills training for doctors, but anyone involved in people-work will appreciate the need to have this sensitivity developed. It is one of the distinctive features of this dictionary that such themes are given detailed treatment: this is one of many areas where practitioners feel the need for guidance and encouragement, and which are often missing from some of the standard textbooks.

There is always a danger, admittedly, of giving the impression that there is only one right way of dealing with issues. When it comes to agency guidelines and procedures, of course, practitioners need to know what to do and what course of action to follow. But with the rich tapestry of communication skills, it would be far from helpful to give the suggestion that we are trying to clone people into certain behaviours. There is nothing worse than being dealt with by someone who seems to be on 'auto-pilot' and who deals with us mechanistically, without that essential spark of warm humanity. This book has a different aim altogether. It seeks to encourage the practitioner, at whatever stage they may be in their careers as people-workers, to use the entries as *pictures* and as *mirrors*. When we look at a picture, we should be drawn into it, and be able to appreciate both the overall story it seeks to communicate, and also some of the fine detail that is important to the theme. It helps us to learn, and to widen our appreciation. In a mirror, however, we see ourselves as we are, and this helps us appreciate ways in which we need to change and develop to improve our practice. There is a constant implicit theme throughout the book: *how will you handle issues in such a way that you can make these skills part of the 'real you' as a practitioner, so that they have an integrity and genuineness about them when you are working with someone else?* One thing you can be sure of: people will pick up very quickly whether you are conveying genuine human interest, care and concern, or whether you are simply 'going through the motions'.

It is very easy, unfortunately, to hide behind the professional practitioner role. To do your job effectively, it is important that you fulfil this professional role properly because it highlights what you can and cannot do with and for the other person. You will want to come across as caring and friendly, but you are not there to be a friend. Your role is both time-limited and task-orientated: when the job is done, you must end the relationship and close the file. What happens afterwards is not your concern. But hiding behind the role is a different story. This is when you do the job automatically, and with little warmth. You seem 'dead behind the eyes', as if you do not really care about what you are doing and you fall into the trap that divides the world into two groups. First, the professional, trained helpers who are the experts; they know what they are doing and are competent in their roles, and should be treated with respect and gratitude, come what may, by those who fall into the second group. These are the unfortunate ones, who are problem-laden, inadequate and unable to cope, who need help and support, and who would quickly 'go under' were it not for the service which the professionals provide. Such attitudes lead to arrogance, and undermine the essential value base of people-work that celebrates the dignity, value and worth of each and every human being. It also denies the fact that, in their personal lives, many professional practitioners experience the full range of turmoil, failure and incompetence as does anyone else. Also, many people who approach professionals for help and support display a far greater ability to cope and have deeper resources of resilience than is often realised. The helping relationship, therefore, that communication skills are there to facilitate, needs a measure of humility, human warmth and genuineness that respects the common humanity that we all share, and a willingness to respect and enhance the determination that other people display in tackling the problems and difficulties which beset them.

To hide behind the professional role also carries the danger of 'taking over'. However satisfying it may feel to do something for the other person – and there will be occasions when this is wholly appropriate – in the end the real 'litmus test' of our work is the extent to which the other person becomes more able to take responsibility for their own life. This is not a re-working of the tired maxim to encourage people 'to stand on their own two feet'. Society is structured in such a complex way these days that the pressures which undermine people's capacity and resilience are ever increasing. It is, however, a reflection of the value base of people-work that respects the dignity of each individual and the strengths we all have to a greater or lesser degree. If your professional help and support can trigger a range of resources, both internal and external, to facilitate this enhanced capacity to cope, your role is validated, but to do this there has to be a valued, effective professional relationship between you.

## LEVELS OF SKILL

The issue of levels of skill is an important dimension to this theme. Trevithick (2012) discusses the journey from basic, through intermediate, to advanced skills which social workers, and indeed all people-workers, will need to take in order to maximise their effectiveness. There are basic foundational skills, such as knowing how and when to use open and closed questions, and how to begin to forge a professional relationship, that need to be introduced to students on their education and training courses so that they can develop a basic level of confidence before they are 'let loose' on the general public. Such is the nature of people-work, however, that it is not possible to plan your progress through a set of increasingly complex stages of communication skills. A surgeon needs to do this: you would not wish to have a complete novice undertake highly complex operations: a gradual progression through the range of medical knowledge and skills is essential, with each stage needing to be effectively accomplished before taking on more advanced work. Similarly in nursing there will be technical levels of expertise which you will gain and develop as your career progresses. In any professional people-work there will be more complex areas which, as Woodcock Ross (2011) clearly demonstrates, demand greater experience and expertise before you can begin to undertake them: child protection, complex mental health work, specialist advice and tribunal work are examples that spring to mind. Generalist skills, therefore, need to be enriched by a set of specialist knowledge and skills for such work to be undertaken successfully.

But when it comes to the generalist skills relating to communication with people, it is far from straightforward. There is no guarantee, for example, that a relative 'beginner' will not find themselves thrown in at the deep end. The interview that seems on paper to be simple and straightforward may suddenly take you into unchartered territory of complexity, where sensitive communication is all important. This illustrates the dilemma that supervisors and practice educators have when selecting work for an inexperienced student: you never know what is going to happen! The approach taken in this dictionary, therefore, does not seek to give each entry a 'complexity rating'; it takes for granted that the level to which you will be able to go with the person depends upon two interweaving factors: your skills at exploring issues, and the person's willingness to trust you and to go deeper.

A relatively inexperienced worker, for example, could establish a basic level of communication with the other person, and deal effectively with what sometimes is called the 'presenting problem'. This may seem straightforward enough, and may be dealt with very quickly. The real skill comes in working out whether or not the 'real' reason for the person coming to you is much deeper and more complex. Being able to explore this possibility requires a great level of sensitivity that some workers have 'in spades' from day one, while with others it takes time to develop. So the new student who is very sensitive might find that they are uncovering much deeper issues than either they or their supervisor suspected were there, *precisely because* they had the ability to explore and probe sensitively. By contrast, a worker who has not developed this capacity might find that they are getting through their caseload in double-quick time simply because they are not able to reach a deeper level.

There is no 'cut and dried' route to success in this: it almost always depends upon the indefinable quality of the 'chemistry' between the worker and the other person, and the extent to which they have been able to develop a trusting relationship together. Without that, the interview is likely to remain at a relatively superficial level. But even for an excellent worker there can be pitfalls: the other person may 'put the shutters up'; factors to do with age, 'race', gender and class may prove far more influential upon the outcome than had been realised. This is what makes people-work so fascinating, rewarding, frustrating and at times bewildering, not just at the outset of your career, but all the way through. And it is for this reason that reflective practice and supervision are so essential to you throughout your career. You need always to be looking into the mirror of reflective practice to ensure that you are always giving of your best and are using your communication skills to the best effect.

Each entry in this book therefore may be utilised by both the novice and the 'old hand': all that is needed is the professional openness and willingness to be continually evaluating and improving your practice with the constant oscillation between getting the basics right and pushing back the boundaries of your expertise.

## HOW BEST TO USE THIS BOOK

For it to be most effective and useful, this book needs to be regarded as a working tool that can be quickly and easily accessed, as well as being an encouragement to a more in-depth reflection. However it is used, it seeks to recognise and strengthen your commitment as a practitioner to develop your communication skills, and to be a working companion in your journey towards professional excellence.

The dictionary approach enables you to go straight to the topic or theme that interests you. You will gain a brief overview by reading through each topic, but because communication skills are not to be seen in isolation from each other, you will be signposted to some related concepts dealt with elsewhere in the book to broaden and deepen your knowledge and understanding.

Suggestions for further reading are provided to help you engage with topics in greater depth. The focus in this book is on communication skills: it is not a dictionary of social work, for example, where some of the theoretical concepts would be discussed in great detail. This book is designed to help you 'operationalise' these concepts, not to provide you with a complete discussion of their complexity.

For this reason, considerable emphasis has been placed upon offering activities throughout the book. These have been designed both as individual activities and as group exercises. The book is also designed to be a resource for practice educators, supervisors, mentors, academic teachers and trainers to use as part of their training and teaching programmes. You may well be asked therefore to study a particular entry and to complete the individual or group activity(ies) relevant to that theme in preparation for your next supervision or group training event. To use the book in this way will deeply enrich your learning.

## A NOTE FOR NURSES

Nurses using this book will find much of the content is as relevant to nursing as it is to social work and other professions. All nurses, whether student, associate or qualified, must always work within their scope of practice and ensure that they practise in line with the requirements of the Code (NMC, 2018b). Each chapter of the book will signpost you therefore to sections of the Code to enable you to consider your professional practice and development.

## OUR UNIQUE SELLING POINT (USP)

One of the distinctive features of this book is that special care has been taken to provide guidance and exercises on topics or themes which do not appear in some of the other books on the market. Breaking Bad News, Chairing Meetings, Talks and Presentations, 'tapping' and exploring religious and spiritual issues as part of professional practice are some of the topics where a more detailed treatment is justified in order to maximise the usefulness of the book. For many of the topics there are parallel discussions elsewhere in the literature to which you will be signposted through further reading, enabling this book to offer a more succinct approach. Where we feel we are breaking new ground, however, we have given more space to the discussion. But this is not to suggest that word length is the only indicator of importance. Far from it!

## FINAL THOUGHTS

We hope that this book will become 'well-thumbed' as a valued travelling companion in your professional practice. But the ultimate test of its usefulness will be the extent to which you commit yourself to engage with the issues raised so that the quality of the professional relationships with the people you work with is enhanced. Travel well and practise better!

## REFERENCES

Nursing & Midwifery Council (NMC) (2018a) *The Code: Professional Standards of Practice and Behaviour for Nurses, Midwives and Nursing Associates.* London: NMC.
Nursing & Midwifery Council (NMC) (2018b) *Future Nurse: Standards of proficiency for registered nurses.* London: NMC.
Trevithick, P. (2012) *Social Work Skills: A Practice Handbook*, 3rd edition. Maidenhead: Open University Press.
Woodcock Ross, J. (2011) *Specialist Communication Skills for Social Workers: Focusing on Service Users' Needs.* Basingstoke: Palgrave Macmillan.

# ACCEPTANCE

'Acceptance' is a term which has entered the common parlance of people-work, not least through the seminal works of Rogers (1951), Egan (2017) and Truax and Carkhuff (2007), each of whom emphasised the importance of the personal relationship between the counsellor/worker and the 'client' in a helping relationship. They argued that it is only when a person seeking help believes that they are being accepted for who they are, without being put down or being judged, that any real progress towards change can be achieved. Upon these foundations, the increasingly complex disciplines of counselling and other people-work disciplines have been built (Nelson-Jones, 2014).

The roots of this approach run deep within western philosophy, and also draw particular strength from the monotheistic traditions of Christianity, Judaism and Islam, where the uniqueness of each individual and their accountability to a divine creator is a central tenet of faith. In some ways the current, postmodern fascination with spirituality is highlighting the same point, that each individual seeks their own deep sense of meaning and purpose, which deserves to be respected and valued by others.

Counselling, of course, is a discrete discipline, even though some of its skills are used by other professional groups. Counselling is not social work, any more than social work is counselling. But the key tenet of acceptance, so vital to counselling, has also become part of the value base and codes of conduct not only of social work but of many other helping professions. It emphasises the importance and uniqueness of each and every person with whom the professional worker comes into contact, and their right to expect to be treated with dignity and respect.

All of this, however, is easier said than done. The big question for any worker is how to put this basic tenet of a professional value base into practice when faced with people whose behaviour is oppressive, abusing and damaging to others. Professional people-workers are called upon daily to work with people whose lifestyles blatantly contradict this value base; their victims testify to their inhumanity. The one thing that acceptance is *not* is any sense of approval for behaviour that demeans and damages others. It is part of the responsibility of people-work professionals to protect those who are vulnerable and at risk in society, and this necessarily involves challenging those who behave oppressively towards others.

It is this tension between these two aspects of our professional value base – acceptance of each individual as unique and precious, and the protection of the vulnerable from abuse – which places this theme firmly in the arena of communication skills. It is arguably one of the most difficult skills to develop for any worker, not least because our sense of moral outrage at some people's behaviour will seep into our dealings with them, however scrupulous we are with the language we use in our interviews and discussions.

## Activity

To illustrate this point, imagine for a moment you have to interview or nurse someone who has committed a heinous offence against a vulnerable child or older person. The graphic details of their behaviour are outlined in your file and you feel physically sickened that someone could do this sort of thing to another human being. Just spend a few moments by yourself or with others whom you trust, quietly imagining yourself face to face with this person, and identify the feelings which are churning around inside you, and what you would like to do to them if you had them alone in a dark alley. It could, after all, have been your child, your parent or grandparent.

And now get in touch with how these feelings are manifesting themselves in how you are sitting – your facial expressions, the tenseness of your body language; how your fists so easily become clenched; 'and now I am supposed to accept this person? You must be joking!'

If you have attempted this Activity honestly, you will find yourself firmly in this tension-filled territory which has already been described. Your professional value base insists that you treat this individual with dignity and respect; your own humanity rebels against what they have done. It is precisely because of this tension, however, that codes of conduct have been drawn up to ensure that we do not allow our own feelings and (let it be said) our prejudices to get in the way of the tasks which society expects of us. The significance of the Activity you have just completed is its power to remind you how strong your feelings can be, and to make the point that, whether you like it or not, those feelings will be communicated to a greater or lesser extent to the person with whom you are seeking to work. In other words, you may be able to use all the appropriate words in your interview but the high emotions of how you are *really* feeling will seep out rather like a bad smell, and will pervade and strongly influence how the other person responds. They will then respond not so much to your words but to your non-verbal communication, and that gives them a very clear message: you are *not* accepted.

## WAYS FORWARD

The discussion so far has aimed at uncovering, as honestly as we can, the way we sometimes feel about those whom we are seeking to help or look after. The following pointers to best practice are offered to help you begin to deal with this particularly difficult area.

### Supervision and preparation

If you know you are going to have to deal with a situation that stirs up strong feelings in you, it is imperative that you prepare properly. This includes talking through with a trusted supervisor, manager, ward sister or practice educator, how you feel about this particular scenario, and being honest about your feelings. You will find, more often than not, that this discussion will help you put things into perspective and enable you to deal with the person professionally. To know that you have a safe place in which to deal with *your* feelings will enable you to provide a safe place for the other person to deal with theirs. It also opens up the possibility that your supervisor may feel that someone else should take over responsibility for this case. For example, if it has triggered off within you some deep-seated hurt which cannot be easily resolved, then it would be better for someone else to handle this particular referral.

## Accept yourself

Acceptance is not just how you treat other people: it has a dimension to it that involves how you think of yourself. We all have our strengths and our weaknesses; things we are good at and things we struggle with; our personal victories and our individual wounds. The best people-workers are often those who have come to a deep understanding and acceptance of who they are, warts and all, and who reach out to others not from a position of moral superiority, but from their shared humanity. Yes, we may abhor what some people have done to hurt others, but few of us as people-workers have been able to avoid hurting people in our own relationships. The sense of our own frailty and capacity to be unloving and uncaring, however, can be channelled into a more humble approach in our work with others, and help us realise that we all struggle with trying to make a success of our lives.

## Remember to practise the basics

Your basic communication skills training is there, not only for you to fall back on but to use as an essential strategy in offering acceptance to another person. The way you introduce yourself; your tone of voice; your non-verbal communication skills; your active listening skills – all are there to be used to help put the person at their ease. They will then begin to feel that this is a space and time for them, so that no matter what they have done they are being listened to and accepted in a respectful and dignified manner.

## Be honest

Even if the person you are working with shows no remorse for their actions, you can still legitimately raise with them how many people in society (and by implication you too) feel about how they have behaved. It is perfectly legitimate to be clear with people that their actions have damaged others and that part of your role is to help protect vulnerable people. Importantly, if they can see you as an ally to help them change their behaviour, and begin to realise that in your acceptance of them as an individual you are opening up the possibility of a changed lifestyle, you will have done them an immeasurable service. To demonstrate a belief that the person can change is perhaps one of the most important messages you can ever communicate.

### Be focused

As with all people-work, you will need to communicate clearly with the person you are working with why you are involved; how you can agree in partnership with them what needs to be achieved, and how this will be effected; and also what the consequences are likely to be if progress is not achieved. Accepting the *consequences* of a person's behaviour is as important as accepting the person themselves.

## CELEBRATE DIVERSITY

So far, the discussion has focused on a particularly sharp set of issues that throw into high relief the tension that is inherent in this theme of acceptance. However, it is important now to widen the context in order to demonstrate its relevance to the whole range of people-work. As already noted, the communication skills aspects of the discussion arise from the value base of our work, which may be characterised by the celebration of diversity.

Diversity is, by definition, a complex theme, but in this context it reflects the multicultural, multi-faith and multi-dimensional aspect of society. If racism, sexism, classism, disablism and homophobia are the shadows cast by oppressive world views, then the positive aspect of this is the celebration of society where people and their chosen world views, lifestyles and various differences are both respected and celebrated as being an enrichment of our communities. As before, it is important that you understand the implications of this value base for people-work. You need to explore your own world view and prejudices in an honest and open way, other-wise you may jeopardise the work you seek to undertake.

Here too, however, there are points of tension for people-work practice. Not every world view may be of equal value; some litmus test has to be applied to make judge-ments about whether the behaviours towards others which flow from certain world views are deemed to be respectful or oppressive. In exploring these issues, however, the same approach as we outlined above needs to be adopted, and the same com-munication skills implemented, to demonstrate that acceptance is not an empty theoretical perspective but rather a commitment and an energy which pervades all our communication with others.

### Group exercise

The issue of mercy killing raises profound moral, ethical, personal and professional issues. The story of Kay Gildergale who helped to end the life of her seriously ill daughter, for example, is particularly challenging. To help you explore this further, you will need to research some examples that have been to court. With the help of your tutor, debate the issues and see if you can identify what are the key moral and legal themes to emerge.

## FINAL THOUGHTS

This discussion has shown how a topic like acceptance, which is fundamental to the value base of much people-work, pervades every aspect of communication skills. It is not a neat, self-contained concept: indeed, the ease with which it can be defined belies the challenge that is inherent within it for all people-work practice. It raises for you, in all your work, both in the preparation, delivery and evaluation of your engagement with others, the powerful question of whether the person you have been working with really feels accepted as a result of your intervention. There is possibly no greater challenge.

## REFERENCES AND FURTHER READING

Bach, S. and Grant, A. (2015) *Communication and Interpersonal Skills for Nursing*, 3rd edition. Exeter: Learning Matters.

Egan, G. (2017) *The Skilled Helper: A Client Centred Approach*, 2nd edition. Boston, MA: Cengage.

Hugman, B. (2009) *Health Care Communication*. London: Pharmaceutical Press.

Mearns, D. and Thorne, B. (2013) *Person-Centred Counselling in Action*, 4th edition. London: Sage.

Nelson-Jones, R. (2014) *Theory and Practice of Counselling and Therapy*, 6th edition. London: Sage.

Rogers, C.R. (1951) *Client-Centred Therapy*. Boston, MA: Houghton Mifflin.

Trevithick, P. (2012) *Social Work Skills: A Practice Handbook*, 3rd edition. Maidenhead: Open University Press.

Truax, C.B. and Carkhuff, R.R. (2007) *Towards Effective Counseling and Psychotherapy: Training and Practice*. Somerset, NJ: Aldine/Transaction.

**RELATED CONCEPTS** active listening; anti-discriminatory practice; counselling; non-verbal communication; reflective practice; spirituality

**ENGAGING WITH THE PCF** diversity; skills and interventions; knowledge; values and ethics

**ENGAGING WITH THE NMC CODE** prioritise people; promote professionalism and trust

## Service user snippet

Tom (65), currently serving a prison sentence for child abuse:

'I was dreading meeting the prison chaplain: I was so ashamed and scared. But without condoning what I had done she seemed really to care about me as me. I can't tell you how great that felt.'

# ACTIVE LISTENING

Active listening ensures that everything that a person is trying to say is fully received and understood by the listener. This includes attempting to understand not just what the person is saying with their chosen words, but what some of their underlying thoughts and feelings are, which may be conveyed as much by what they do *not* say and by their body language, as by the words they use.

The term 'active listening' is frequently used by helping professionals to underline the importance of this activity. It has several layers to it, and it is not merely hearing the words that are being spoken.

Active listening is, of course, easier said than done, which is why such an emphasis is laid upon it as a core communication skill. To illustrate its complexity, undertake the following Activity either by yourself, with a companion or in a small group.

## Activity

See how many different tones of voice you can use in saying the words 'Can I help you?'. You will quickly discover that some tones of voice can contradict the words you are using, just as a very defensive body posture can have a similar effect.

This is what is sometimes called the 'music behind the words' – and it is the music that conveys the *real* meaning of what is being communicated. If the listener takes the words simply at face value, the real meaning could be ignored.

Of course, you may speculate why this should be so, and the reason may vary from person to person. What this Activity illustrates is that communication is a complex activity, and that if you are going to work successfully with people, your whole being must be attuned to what is being said.

It goes without saying that in any interaction with someone you are seeking to support, nurse or work with, you need to be clear about what you are trying to do. The listening skills that you need will vary according to the nature of the task. For example, if you are a welfare rights worker doing a benefits check for someone, you will certainly need to adopt a caring, understanding approach throughout, but for much of the interview you will be gathering and interpreting factual information which you need to help you calculate their eligibility for particular benefits. In a similar way, a doctor or nurse may need to elicit crucial information about a patient's symptoms in order to reach an accurate diagnosis. A social worker or probation officer preparing a court report will need to elicit and interpret information about a person's behaviour. By contrast, a counsellor working with a deeply distressed person following a major loss in their life will be focusing heavily on that person's feelings, and will be exploring a very sensitive aspect of their life, which requires a different set of skills as they seek to explore and develop that person's self-awareness. Someone who is working with people whose relationships are breaking down will use the skills of trying to help each of them understand what the other is saying, and use interpretative skills to a considerable degree to help people who have become deaf to each other to begin to hear each other's 'music' once more.

These examples illustrate the complexity of the listening task. One common theme, however, is the type of questions that can be used in active listening. These are commonly grouped together into two categories: open questions and closed questions.

*Open questions* are used when you want to help someone 'open up' about themselves, to give you some insights into how they are feeling, or to explore a situation in more depth. They do not allow a straightforward 'yes' or 'no' response, but instead invite the person to talk about the topic. For example:

- Can you tell me how this happened?
- What did your parents think about …?
- Can you tell me in your own words about …?
- Why do you think that was?

Some people discourage the use of the 'why?' question as being too threatening; it can put people 'on the spot' and may make conversation more difficult, especially if it assumes that a measure of blaming is implicit or even explicit in the question ('*Why* on earth did you do that?'). But good communication skills are not about slavishly following a set of rules with their 'dos and don'ts': they are about developing your own style, and realising that with sensitivity and appropriate voice tones you can encourage people to open up and share their story with you.

It is your sensitivity that is all-important. Not everyone will feel able to 'open up' easily and share their deep thoughts and feelings. Some need to go step by step, and to be led by the interviewer cautiously until they gain the confidence to go deeper. This is why closed questions also have such an important role to play.

*Closed questions* invite a straightforward 'yes' or 'no' answer ('Did you hit him?'), and are necessary in gathering factual information in as straightforward a way as possible. Closed questions can give a message to the interviewee that you are in charge, know what you are doing and where you are going, and that they can put their confidence in you.

It is certainly not the case that open questions are good and closed questions bad: that is a gross caricature. Each has its part to play in a well-balanced effective interview, and it is up to you to judge which of them will be most appropriate and effective as the interview unfolds.

## BASIC SKILLS

The complexity of active listening is well illustrated by Trevithick (2012: 172), who lists 20 basic skills involved in listening. These are:

1  Being as open, intuitive, empathetic and self-aware as possible.
2  Maintaining good eye contact.
3  Having an open and attentive body orientation or posture.
4  Paying attention to non-verbal forms of communication and meaning.
5  Allowing for and using silence as a form of communication.
6  Taking up an appropriate physical distance.
7  Picking up and following cues.
8  Being aware of our own distracting mannerisms and behaviour.
9  Avoiding vague, unclear and ambiguous comments.
10  Being aware of the importance of people finding their own words in their own time.
11  Remembering the importance of the setting and the general physical environment.
12  Minimising the possibility of interruptions and distractions.
13  Being sensitive to the overall mood of the interview, including what is not being communicated.
14  Listening for the emotional content of the interview and adapting questions as appropriate.
15  Checking out and seeking feedback wherever possible and appropriate.
16  Being aware of the importance of timing, particularly where strong feelings are concerned.
17  Remembering the importance of tone, particularly in relation to sensitive or painful issues.
18  Avoiding the dangers of preconceptions, stereotyping or labelling, or making premature judgements or evaluations.
19  Remembering to refer to theories that are illuminating and helpful, and also, where appropriate, to explain, in an accessible language, theories that may aid understanding.
20  Being as natural, spontaneous and relaxed as possible.

Put like that, listening skills may seem daunting, even impossible to get completely right. They are a challenge, and it sometimes needs a list like that to remind us that to listen actively can be one of the hardest tasks we ever undertake.

### Group exercise

With the help of your tutor or supervisor, go through the 20 skills listed above. Try to think of examples for each one and, as a group, explore ways of how you would take account of these active listening skills in practice. Include an open discussion around any different dialects within your group and cultural differences around making eye contact and body language, and what impact this may make upon your practice.

## SUMMARISING

Summarising is a useful skill, which helps to check the pace and progress of an interview. Essentially, this means taking some time out from the actual flow of the interview and trying to put into words the story so far as you perceive it. This serves several useful functions:

- It demonstrates to the interviewee that you have been listening to what they are saying and that you have grasped the main issues clearly.
- It provides the interviewee with an opportunity to confirm the accuracy of your summary and (importantly) to put right any misunderstanding you may have developed.
- It facilitates the process of empathy between you and the interviewee.
- It provides a structured staging post in the interview to take stock and to decide how to move on to the next stage.
- It is also a useful technique to use when the interview 'runs into the sand' and you need to 'get unstuck'.

Obviously, in the course of an interview lasting, say, for an hour, you will not want to use this summarising technique too often as that would become tedious and mechanistic. Perhaps two or three times, including the summary you will want to offer at the very end of the interview, will normally be about right.

## PARAPHRASING

This is a similar skill to summarising, but it provides a narrower focus in that you can use it frequently to 'mirror' or reflect back to the interviewee a particular thought, concept or feeling they are trying to express. This skill involves putting into your own words what you think the other person is trying to express. This has several advantages:

- It enables you to show that you have been listening to the interviewee.
- It provides an opportunity for the interviewee to confirm, or adjust, the feedback you have provided.
- It helps to establish empathy.
- It provides an opportunity for the interviewee to see themselves in the 'verbal mirror' you have provided as a stimulus for further reflection.

However, as with all 'techniques', it is important that they are used sensitively and not 'robotically': that would be extremely frustrating and counter-productive. The interviewee may end up feeling that they cannot get it right because you are always changing what they have said into something 'more acceptable to you', and that is the last message you will want to convey. Use the technique, therefore, if you get stuck, or feel that the other person is struggling, or you feel you need their help to understand them better.

## CLARIFYING

It will come as no surprise to you to discover that people cannot always easily put into words what they are feeling or what they need to tell you. If you need any confirmation of this statement, look no further than yourself. Think back to an occasion when you were deeply upset or distressed and had to talk to someone. The chances are that all your usual confidence and articulacy somehow drained away, and you were left groping for the words that might express how you felt.

There will be occasions in an interview, therefore, where it is likely that you will not understand what is being said, for whatever reason. The skills of clarifying are important, because you do not want to get to the end of a long complex interview and still feel in the dark about some key issues and facts.

The important thing to remember here is that the interviewee will be doing their very best to communicate clearly, often under difficult circumstances. So you do not want to give out a message that they are 'making a hash' of it. Instead, it is important that *you* take responsibility for not fully understanding, and ask them to help you to gain the fuller picture. As is so often the case in interviewing, you need to find a form of words that feels right to you: there is no magic mantra which will always work. But something like the following may be helpful to start you off in your search for your own best approach:

> 'J, you have given me a very clear picture of how upset all this has made you feel. I wonder if you can help me with some of the details which I'm afraid I have not been able to sort out in my own mind yet.'

> 'Gosh J, this is a very difficult situation – no wonder you feel so …; I wonder if you could help me understand a bit better about 'x'?'

> 'J, this is like a jigsaw – you have explained very clearly about 'x' and 'y', but I need your help please to understand about 'z' and how this fits into the overall picture.'

> 'J, I wonder if it would help if we put some of the things you have told me up here on the flip chart – it would certainly help me get a better picture.'

You might also find that the use of a genogram or an ecomap is a good way of clarifying the situation.

## FURTHER ISSUES

There are additional complexities to be taken into account. They may be stated briefly but each of these issues deserves detailed consideration and reflection. The issues are gender, age, race and disability.

### Gender

The impact of gender must not be overlooked. For some people, and within certain cultures, it is of great importance that women have the opportunity to talk with a female worker, just as in medical matters many women prefer to have a female GP. Similarly, in some cultures, a man would want to be able to talk things over with a male worker. But even if there are not cultural imperatives to consider, this dimension will always be present, and it is important that, as a worker, you think about what impact this will have upon each professional encounter you experience. There will be occasions when you need to raise this issue specifically with the other person so that it can be appropriately addressed and not allowed to fester.

## Age

There is no denying that ageism can sometimes undermine a relationship you are trying to develop. For example, a very young worker at the beginning of their career may meet with a much older person who may be tempted to disregard their expertise and potential effectiveness simply on the grounds of age and assumed inexperience. By contrast, a much older worker, when trying to work with a younger person, may find that they represent a parent figure so strongly that the young person 'puts up the shutters' and refuses to have anything to do with them. There are no easy ways around this. Sometimes it is a question of how 'cases' are allocated within an agency. What is important, however, is that you will need to raise these issues directly and try to talk about the 'blocks' that are being put up, in the hope that by airing them they can gradually be removed, and a trusting relationship established. That will be a challenge to your communication skills admittedly, but until the 'block' is identified it will not be possible to move forward.

## Race

One of the tenets of anti-racist practice is that, ideally, people should be able to have a worker from a similar ethnic background to themselves, to help ensure that they are fully 'heard' and that a totally sensitive assessment is made. This involves being aware that for many black and minority ethnic people to go to a predominantly white agency carries the risk of a continuation of racist attitudes and behaviours. However welcoming an agency may try to be with multicultural welcome posters on display, the reality of only being able to offer a white worker can be worrying for a member of a minority ethnic group in this country. It is important to state clearly that this fear or misgiving will have been based on previous experiences of living in a racist community, so the onus must be upon a white worker to acknowledge these issues in a sensitive way, and to check out how best to proceed. There are many examples where this 'checking out' has led to a reduction in mistrust and misgivings, and a good working relationship has subsequently been established with good outcomes. The crucial thing, however, is for white workers to be honest about the issues; to acknowledge that it can be difficult for a predominantly white agency to provide sensitive and appropriate services; and to take the initiative in talking about these issues at the first meeting.

It must also be said, however, that workers from minority ethnic groups can sometimes experience racist behaviour from white people seeking to use the service, and who express resentment that they cannot be seen by a white worker. This calls for strong anti-discriminatory policies by the agency to support all their staff and to make it clear that all members of staff are committed to delivering the best possible service to everyone who needs it. It should also be noted that discriminatory behaviour towards staff should not be tolerated.

## Disability

All organisations need to ensure that their services are disability-friendly. This means that those who seek to use the services of the agency must be able to fully access them, and that the agency must also be a disability-friendly employer. There are, of course, some particular challenges, for both staff and users of the service, when working with people who are Deaf or hard of hearing, people who have communication difficulties, or are visually impaired. It is important that due consideration is given to these issues so that people are not marginalised and excluded from services.

---

### Group exercise

Spend some time thinking what the challenges are for communication skills in regard to the four issues outlined above – gender, age, race, disability – for your particular service or agency.

---

## Language, dialect and culture

One further set of issues deserves to be added to the list of complexities for active listening skills. It is best practice that people who wish to access services should be able to do so in their language of choice. This will mean that, on occasion, you will need to negotiate for a skilled professional interpreter to be present for your interviews so that information can be accurately exchanged. Your agency should be able to access interpreter services in your area. This includes British Sign Language for people who are Deaf. Somewhat more complicated, however, is the issue of dialects, especially if you are new to an area and are unfamiliar both with the music of the local dialect and some of the words and phrases that, for local people, enrich their sense of identity, but which can significantly disempower a worker seeking to accurately communicate with them. There is no substitute for seeking out some local people who would be willing to spend some time with you, helping you to become attuned to the dialect and giving you a glossary of common terms that are used. But until you are comfortable, you will need to develop the skill of asking sensitively for explanations and translations, in a way which makes it clear that it is *you* who are on the learning curve: it is not the other person's fault! There are also important issues to consider around intercultural awareness, and some of the 'messages' that white people, for example, may (however unwittingly) give to members of minority ethnic communities that may imply racist or stereotypical attitudes.

---

## Group exercise

What are the issues around language, culture and dialect in your area? How are you dealing with these? Can you prepare a glossary for new members of staff or students joining your team? Or perhaps make this into a student project?

---

## FINAL THOUGHTS

Active listening skills are complex, but they are the fundamental bedrock of good practice. They cannot be taken for granted. They need to be worked at, and as we have seen, some of the issues you will need to explore and deal with may be particularly challenging. But without good listening skills, your people-work career will never get past first base.

## REFERENCES AND FURTHER READING

Allen, G. and Langford, D. (2007) *Effective Interviewing in Social Work and Social Care: A Practice Guide.* Basingstoke: Palgrave Macmillan.

Bach, S. and Grant, A. (2015) *Communication and Interpersonal Skills for Nursing,* 3rd edition. Exeter: Learning Matters.

Hargie, O. (2016) *Skilled Interpersonal Communication,* 6th edition. Hove: Routledge.

Hugman, B. (2009) *Health Care Communication.* London: Pharmaceutical Press.

Koprowska, J. (2019) *Communication and Interpersonal Skills in Social Work,* 5th edition. Exeter: Learning Matters.

Ryde, J. (2009) *Being White in the Helping Professions: Developing Effective Intercultural Awareness.* London: Jessica Kingsley.

Thompson, N. (2011) *Effective Communication,* 2nd edition. Basingstoke: Palgrave Macmillan.

Thompson, N. (2015) *People Skills,* 4th edition. Basingstoke: Palgrave Macmillan.

Trevithick, P. (2012) *Social Work Skills: A Practice Handbook,* 3rd edition. Maidenhead: Open University Press.

Woodcock Ross, J. (2016) *Specialist Communication Skills: Developing Professional Capability,* 2nd edition. London: Palgrave.

**RELATED CONCEPTS** acceptance; dealing with upset service users; ecomaps; empathy; genograms; getting unstuck; interpreters

**ENGAGING WITH THE PCF** acceptance; ecomaps; empathy; genograms; getting unstuck

**ENGAGING WITH THE NMC CODE** prioritise people

### Service user snippet

Fran (37), mental health service user:

'For the first time in my life I felt as if someone had really listened to me and heard the real me inside ... I can't tell you what a relief that was.'

# ADVISING

Across the wide spectrum of people-work, advice-giving – or advising – receives frequent mention, either in terms of what the organisation offers to those who use its services, or in terms of what is definitely not on offer. In counselling, for example, and in organisations such as the Samaritans, there is a strong ethos against giving advice. For this range of people-work, giving advice can be counter-productive: it smacks of telling people what to do, of making people's decisions for them or pointing them in certain directions, with the implicit assumption that the professional knows best. In counselling, therefore, the worker's role is to help the person being counselled to think through the issues and the likely consequences of any decisions they take, and to decide on the course of action that they feel is best for them, and for which they, and they alone, can take responsibility.

By contrast, there are other organisations and professional people-workers where advice-giving is their raison d'être. If we need to understand some legal, technical, medical or financial matters, we naturally go to those people who have accredited expertise and who can explain things to us, and advise us accordingly. Any decisions remain ours to take, but they will be taken in the light of professional advice we have received from appropriate experts, upon whose judgement and advice we rely, and against whom we can apply for legal compensation if their advice is at fault.

In between are a range of people-workers, such as social workers, youth and community workers and probation officers, whose role may include an advice-giving element (e.g. welfare benefits advice) alongside a combination of care and control responsibilities. Decisions about people's lives may sometimes have to be taken against their express wishes, in order either to safeguard themselves or to protect vulnerable people and children in their care. In such scenarios, a social worker may well advise someone about their rights, but will still take their child into care if that is deemed necessary.

Having said that, there is a tendency in some people-workers to jump in too quickly and to tell people what to do before really listening to their story. It may make the people-worker feel better, but the service user may feel they haven't been listened to properly or that someone else has taken over from them in an early rush to solve problems. The rule of thumb therefore is listen first; *advise only if necessary.*

Alongside all of this is the ever-increasing independent advice sector represented by such organisations as AdviceUK and Citizens Advice, agencies that deliver advice through a nationwide network of advice centres to anyone who needs free, confidential and impartial advice across a wide range of issues, including welfare benefits, debt, housing, immigration and employment. These core services are delivered by professionally trained staff, supported by supervised volunteers who operate a triage service and deliver low-level advice. Some work is commissioned by the Legal Aid

Agency. Welfare rights and other forms of advice are also commonly made available in social services departments and in a range of healthcare settings.

This brief overview indicates the complexity of advice and advice-giving services, and highlights the difficulty in providing a succinct definition of what advice is. Robson and Savage from Staffordshire University suggest that:

> Advice work can best be described in terms of an alloy, a composite of a range of functions which when welded together form the basis of what is generally described as 'advice work'. (Personal communication)

It is important to recognise that the government has made strenuous efforts in recent years to establish standards for advice-giving. For legal advice work there is the Specialist Quality Mark (SQM), whereas generalist services are covered by the Advice Quality Standard (AQS), audited through the Advice Services Alliance (ASA). Funding for social welfare advice work relies upon a myriad of diverse sources, including government legal aid, although the scope of this was significantly reduced by the Legal Aid, Sentencing and Punishment of Offenders Act 2012. Within this Act a number of advice subject areas, for example debt and employment, were completely removed from legal aid scope.

As far as the communication skills needed for advice work are concerned, Robson and Savage outline the key communication skills needed in advice work:

> Non-verbal skills; active listening, questioning, summarising, paraphrasing, presenting/explaining/interpreting information; checking/clarifying understanding; using the telephone; written skills; letter writing, form filling, presenting of information; negotiation (persuading and influencing) and advocacy (representation–verbal presentation skills). (Personal communication)

The key to advising on social welfare issues relies, as ever, on a full exploration of the issues, looking at the options both legally and tactically so that the client can then make an informed judgement on the best way forward. Usually the options are readily apparent with the adviser providing the required information supported by statutory legislation, policy and case law. In advice work there is no counselling, but support can be provided when the client has decided on certain actions, including representation at hearings. In addition to the provision of advice, advice agencies in the social welfare sector will also undertake social policy work, locally and nationally, through research and campaigns to address social welfare issues affecting larger groups within society.

## Activity

In your current role, what opportunities (if any) are there for giving advice? What sort of advice do you feel able to offer? What organisations would you need to refer people to for more specialist advice?

It will be clear from this discussion that advice-giving uses the full range of communication skills that many other professional helpers use, and that these are essential in order to maintain the high standards of the agencies involved.

---

## Group exercise

With your tutor or supervisor, think of the work you currently undertake. Does your agency have boundaries for any advice provided? Explore other agencies in your area that provide specialist information and advice, and make a list to use and refer to.

---

## FINAL THOUGHTS

Advice-giving is a very specific and professional skill for which appropriate training is required to protect both the advisers and their clients. You need to be very clear therefore about the boundaries in your role as a people-worker, and when it is appropriate and even necessary to refer people on to other better qualified agencies.

## REFERENCES AND FURTHER READING

Child Poverty Action Group (CPA) (2019) *Welfare Benefits and Tax Credits Handbook 2019/2020*. London: Child Poverty Action Group.

Finch, E. and Fanfinski, S. (2017) *Legal Skills*, 6th edition. Oxford: Oxford University Press.

Greaves, I. (2019) *Disability Rights Handbook*, 44th edition. London: Disability Rights UK.

Heslop, E. (2014) *Giving Legal Advice*, 2nd edition. London: Legal Action Group.

Madge, P. (2020) *Debt Advice Handbook*, 13th edition. London: Child Poverty Action Group.

Ministry of Justice (2012) *Legal Aid, Sentencing and Punishment of Offenders Act 2012*, Part 1. Available at www.legislation.gov.uk/ukpga/2012/10/contents (accessed 22/01/2019).

Web resources

AdviceUK – www.adviceuk.org.uk/ (accessed 11/09/2019)

Citizens Advice – www.citizensadvice.org.uk (accessed 11/09/2019)

Legal Aid Agency – www.justice.gov.uk/legal-aid (accessed 11/09/2019)

---

**RELATED CONCEPTS** active listening; advocacy; establishing a professional relationship

**ENGAGING WITH THE PCF** contexts and organisations; skills and interventions; professionalism

**ENGAGING WITH THE NMC CODE** practise effectively; preserve safety

## Service user snippet

Brian (27), homeless and in debt:

'Citizens Advice were fantastic – I was about to top myself but they sorted things out with me and I feel I can face the future now.'

# ADVOCACY

The dictionary definitions of 'advocacy' describe the role as being 'one who pleads the case of another'; in other words, to defend, support, represent and argue positively on behalf of someone else (*Chambers Twentieth Century Dictionary*, 1901). Trevithick (2012: 267) notes that advocacy aims to ensure that the voices and interests of service users are heard and responded to in ways that affect attitudes, policy, practice and service delivery, and that the mandate for this can be found in the objectives of the National Health Service and Community Care Act 1990, which is 'to give people a greater say in how they live their lives and the services they need to help them to do so' (DH, 1990, cited in Trevithick, 2012: 267).

This seemingly straightforward concept does not, however, reflect the complexity of advocacy as an activity which is practised by a range of people-workers and others. For example:

- In court, a solicitor or barrister will advocate on your behalf by providing detailed and sometimes legally complex information and opinion to the magistrate or judge.
- Social workers and health workers will, from time to time, speak up on behalf of their service user, client or patient to support their claim for a particular welfare benefit or a claim to housing.
- A social worker or youth worker may well speak up for a young person who is finding it difficult to find employment, and help them to obtain a job interview.
- A Citizens Advice adviser will represent you and speak on your behalf at a tribunal.
- Someone involved in citizen advocacy may act as a befriender or as an encourager to someone who lacks confidence, perhaps because of emotional difficulties, medical problems or a learning difficulty, and will help them put forward their views.
- A group of people may get together as a self-advocacy group or organisation to help further their cause or to seek an improvement in their circumstances. This is sometimes referred to as 'peer advocacy'.

This spectrum – from the 'hard end' of legal advocacy to the 'softer' informal style – involves, to a degree, all the skills needed for effective advocacy, even though some forms of advocacy may require specific training and experience (e.g. legal advocacy and Citizens Advice work).

# Activity

1   Spend a few moments thinking about a situation where you have been involved in an advo-
    cacy role. Note the main issues involved. What were you called to do? Were there any difficul-
    ties or dilemmas for you? Where do you think the real power lay? What was the outcome of
    the advocacy? How did it make you feel?
2   Think now of an occasion where you have perhaps needed an advocate. How did that make
    you feel? What would be your expectations? How would you define good advocacy and poor
    advocacy? How would each make you feel?

The issues you have identified in the above Activity will form a useful background
to this discussion, and we invite you to refer back to your experience when reflecting
on the issues being raised.

The first point to stress is the importance of being very clear in your own mind
about what the issues are. Without such clarity, you could end up in a complicated
and confused situation. You also need to be clear, when considering your role,
exactly what it is you are being asked to do. Will you be speaking up on behalf of
the person, representing their views and needs, and being their sole mouthpiece? Or
will your role be to facilitate and encourage *them* to do the talking, with you
remaining in the background as a friendly support? In other words, will you be
working for them, or will they be working for themselves, but with your support?

## ETHICAL CONSIDERATIONS

It was made clear in the introduction that any discussion about communication
skills has to include an ethical dimension. Skills are not used in a moral vacuum, but
reflect the values of the person using them. It is important therefore in advocacy
work to ensure that formal communication skills are used within the basic principles of this type of work.

Bateman (1995: 26–41) highlights six main principles for what he describes as
'principled advocacy' which, although drawn from a legal context and using the
legal language of 'clients', are relevant across a wider range of advocacy work. The
six principles are:

1   Act in the client's best interests.
2   Act in accordance with the client's wishes and instructions.
3   Keep the client properly informed.
4   Carry out instructions with diligence and competence.
5   Act impartially and offer frank, independent advice.
6   Maintain rules of confidentiality.

Each of these principles merits detailed discussion and reflection, and you may find
it useful to explore their implications for the situation you analysed in the Activity.

To be an effective advocate, you will need the full range of interpersonal communication skills, linked with a capacity to grasp, at times, complex issues and to formulate and propose solutions. You will need to:

- have the self-confidence to stand up for vulnerable people, and to be willing to stand your ground when challenging organisational bureaucracy;
- be able to interpret complex issues and to help the person you are representing, or whom you are supporting, to understand what is going on, and to be able to produce an effective response;
- accept that sometimes you feel inadequate and powerless against the big battalions, but if you are well prepared and know that you have a strong case to present, then you need to have the courage 'to stick with it'. At such times, your own value base, and your commitment to social justice, will stand you in good stead.

There is a further complex issue that surrounds advocacy, and that concerns power. Everything in the last paragraph is important for the advocate, but it must be tempered with the realisation that power can be seductively 'powerful'. It naturally gives you a good feeling to be powerful; it appeals to your sense of achievement and doing a good job; there is a real 'buzz' when you win a tribunal or gain some advantage for a vulnerable person or family. But there is a risk here: you can too often take over, thereby disempowering those with whom you work. Sometimes it is far more important to spend time empowering others to 'fight their own corner' rather than to rely on the professional 'expert'. These are important considerations when tackling the growing emphasis upon personalisation, enshrined in the Care Act 2014. No longer should welfare professionals feel that they know best: individuals have the right to determine how their resources are best allocated for their wellbeing. Partnership working is therefore at the heart of all good advocacy.

There is, however, a caveat we need to acknowledge here. While is it certainly rewarding for you to take pride in watching people succeed, however falteringly at first, in presenting their own case, it would serve no one's best interests to watch someone flounder towards failure. Part of your skill therefore is to recognise people's strengths and where they would benefit from support, and to negotiate what is the most appropriate strategy.

## Group exercise

With the help of your tutor or supervisor, role play the following scenario. You visit the local housing office with your service user in order to support them applying for temporary accommodation. The housing officer ignores your service user and directs all questions at you. Use the advocacy skills outlined in this chapter to support your service user to self-advocate. As a group, explore the issues arising from the role play, and then give other group members an opportunity to practise their advocacy skills.

# FINAL THOUGHTS

Effective advocacy is perhaps one of the most difficult skills to develop, but arguably one of the most rewarding, in that you are playing a key role not only in helping someone to be fully valued, respected and at times 'rewarded', but also in helping them to gain confidence and to develop assertiveness on their journey towards greater independence.

# REFERENCES AND FURTHER READING

Bateman, N. (1995) *Advocacy Skills: A Handbook for Human Service Professionals*. Aldershot: Ashgate Arena.

Bateman, N. (2000) *Advocacy Skills for Health and Social Care Professionals*. London: Jessica Kingsley.

Boon, A. (1999) *Advocacy*, 2nd edition, Cavendish Legal Skills Series. London: Cavendish Publishing.

Boylan, J. and Dalrymple, J. (2009) *Understanding Advocacy for Children and Young People*. Maidenhead: Open University Press.

Boylan, J. and Dalrymple, J. (2013) *Effective Advocacy in Social Work*. London: Sage.

*Chambers Twentieth Century Dictionary* (1901) London and Edinburgh: W.R. Chambers.

Department of Health (1990) *NHS and Community Care Act*. London: DH.

Department of Health (2014) *Care Act 2014*. London: DH.

Trevithick, P. (2012) *Social Work Skills: A Practice Handbook*, 3rd edition. Maidenhead: Open University Press.

**RELATED CONCEPTS** advising; empowerment, resilience and a strengths perspective

**ENGAGING WITH THE PCF** contexts and organisation; skills and interventions; values and ethics

**ENGAGING WITH THE NMC CODE** prioritise people; preserve safety

Service user snippet

Frankie (21):

'My last worker was rubbish … just left me to get on with things so I nearly lost my flat. This new worker is great – she goes with me to meetings and helps me say what I want.'

# ANTI-DISCRIMINATORY PRACTICE

In all aspects of people-work, anti-discriminatory practice (ADP) not only forms part of the core value base, it also comprises a set of communication skills through which that value base is put into practice. ADP facilitates the celebration of diversity in our complex, multi-layered, multicultural and multi-faith society. ADP skills, therefore, involve cultivating an awareness of how prejudice and oppression operate at various levels in society to certain people's disadvantage, and then actively working to restore the balance so that people get a better opportunity to live full and creative lives. Challenging oppression is an important aspect of ADP and is often referred to directly as anti-oppressive practice (AOP).

In many ways, social work has led the way in our understanding of how ADP is at the heart of best practice, but the basic principles can apply to all aspects of people-work, particularly in the field of health, nursing and social care. One author who has shaped our understanding of ADP is Neil Thompson, whose seminal writing in this area has been hugely influential (see Thompson, 2016, for example). Thompson insists that best practice must take into account three interlocking dimensions to the ways in which prejudice and oppression can operate: the personal (P), the cultural (C) and the structural (S). This theoretical and conceptual framework argues against too-simplistic an understanding of the issues surrounding discrimination. An individual white worker, for example, may strenuously uphold a commitment to anti-racist practice, and this commitment may permeate that worker's individual personal dealings with members of the black community. But this does not alter the fact that at wider levels, in various cultural aspects and in how society is structured, racism is still a powerful, negative force which diminishes black people's life chances. It must be dealt with, therefore, as a fundamental principle of best practice.

## Activity

It is important to take time fully to explore the concept of ADP, and the contribution that the PCS analysis makes to our understanding. Obtain a copy of Thompson's book *Anti-Discriminatory Practice* (2016, 6th edition), and read carefully the first two chapters, where the main themes are explored and discussed. This will give you a firm base upon which to develop your ADP skills.

This PCS analysis provides the framework for exploring the range of skills that are needed to put it into effective practice. Thompson (2016: 10) puts the practice issues succinctly when he states that:

> There is no middle ground; intervention either adds to oppression (or at least condones it) or goes some small way towards easing or breaking such oppressions. In this respect, the political slogan, 'If you are not part of the solution you must be part of the problem', is particularly accurate. An awareness of the sociopolitical context is necessary in order to prevent becoming (or remaining) part of the problem.

This suggests a set of basic questions that you can ask about your professional practice with a service user, enquirer, patient or client. These questions include:

- What are the issues which are clearly under the control or influence of the person you are working with, whether or not you help them?
- To what extent are this person's problems and difficulties due to wider influences, from family, peer group or other cultural groupings?
- How far are this person's difficulties and problems a result of structural issues and influences? Is this individual being blamed or 'pathologised' as a result of these influences?
- What course(s) of action is(are) open to me, and to both of us working in partnership, to tackle some of the wider issues we have identified?

---

### Group exercise

For this exercise you will need to access the Serious Case Review of Child I (Hertfordshire Safeguarding Children Board (2019)), available https://library.nspcc.org.uk/HeritageScripts/Hapi.dll/search2?searchTerm0=C7620 (accessed 16/10/2019). With the help of your tutor or supervisor, explore how Thompson's PCS analysis enables you to develop a deeper understanding of the issues involved.

---

Because ADP is best practice and must therefore permeate all aspects of people-work including nursing, it is difficult to know what issues not to include in this brief introductory discussion. Certainly, key themes such as equality and diversity, empowerment, acceptance and partnership working are all central, as is the use of good active listening skills. The following skills, however, deserve particular mention.

### Non-verbal communication

In a discussion on non-verbal communication, it is important to emphasise that we convey a huge amount of information to another person non-verbally, including our attitude towards them. In a variety of subtle ways, we can convey dislike, disapproval, hostility even, which will be picked up by the other person. They will be made to feel that, for whatever reason, we are being discriminatory, and this may well reinforce other similar messages they have received from society in general. It is imperative, therefore, that from the very first moment of meeting, we convey a genuine warmth and welcome.

## Cultural sensitivity

The service we offer to people needs to be accessible to all members of the community. This is not always easy, of course. Many organisations report that members of minority ethnic communities, or deaf people, for example, do not make use of their services. They can feel alienated and that the service is not for them, in spite of the rhetoric and the multilingual notices of welcome. On occasion, this is a profoundly accurate perception, and organisations need to look long and hard at ways in which they can improve their inclusivity and the 'community ownership' of their service.

On a one-to-one basis, however, cultural sensitivity is an extremely important aspect of ADP. How you greet people; how you handle gender issues; how you acknowledge the differences between you; whether you offer the services of someone who can enable people to use their first language in the interview – these and many other issues are all significant for ADP. No book or training notes can ever cover all aspects of this, of course. It is, however, incumbent upon you to become familiar with the cultural issues of the area in which you work, and to ensure that you make a serious attempt to put cultural sensitivity into practice.

## Personal awareness

Personal awareness is an important aspect of all people-work. It includes our understanding of why we undertake this type of work, what the rewards are and what needs within us are being met by doing it. It also involves being aware of key aspects of ourselves: our age, 'race', gender, class, sexuality, disability, religious background. All of these components make us who we are, and are part of the package of what we communicate to people directly or indirectly when we work with them. Sometimes who we are – our background – will make it easier to work with some people. A shy Asian woman coming into an agency may be hugely relieved to be met by a female Asian worker of a similar age: an immediate rapport may be that much easier to establish. By contrast, a young person may feel that the older worker who is trying to relate to them cannot possibly understand 'where they are coming from', and that the professional in this case represents unwelcome parental and authority figures. The crucial thing for the worker to bear in mind is to be aware of some of these potential advantages and disadvantages, and to be open and honest about them. Sometimes just the act of putting these hesitations into words, and trying to empathise with the other person about these issues, is enough to begin to break down potential barriers to communication.

## Being open and critical about our own practice

The concept of being a reflective practitioner is now well established in people-work, thanks in no small measure to the seminal work of Schön (1983, 1987). This covers a range of issues, including self-awareness and the impact we have upon the people with whom we seek to work. The key point to make here, however, is that the skills of being a reflective practitioner need to be constantly honed and evaluated: there is no guarantee we will get it right. In fact, there is more than an even chance we will get it wrong, to some extent at least. Human diversity and complexity make this almost inevitable. Therefore, we need to have good systems in place to review what we do and how we do it, and to evaluate the impact and outcomes of our work. Supervision is one obvious mechanism for this, particularly if you are still in training, when your practice educator, mentor or supervisor should regularly raise ADP issues with you.

It is also good practice to devise ways of seeking feedback from the service users themselves: they are, after all, the experts in their lives and how you have interacted with them. This is not always straightforward, however. Sometimes people tell you what they think you are hoping to hear! Sometimes their feedback depends upon the extent to which you have been able to deliver what they were hoping to receive. In an era when resources are being cut back, a disappointed service user may reflect that disappointment in the feedback, rather than offer a dispassionate objective evaluation of your practice. But this should not deter you from seeking feedback. Some agencies have a post-event feedback sheet which they send out; or they make a phone call to elicit comments. It is often helpful for a third party to seek this information, such as a supervisor or practice educator. There is no one single, right or best way of seeking this feedback: what is important, however, is that you make it part of your practice to seek it out, and to reflect carefully on what is being said.

## Cultivating the wider picture

An awareness of the PCS analysis should mean that with every piece of work you undertake with someone, these wider perspectives are consciously brought into play. In the discussion about assessment, Thompson's (2012: 119ff) concept of 'helicopter vision' is used precisely to capture the importance of this holistic approach. This ensures that you take into account wider pressures and influences that may have shaped the person's attitudes and behaviour, and also that you draw back from a facile pathologising of a person's problems. Although each and every one of us has a measure of personal responsibility for the world view we have chosen to make sense of our lives and the actions we take, it is often the case that wider pressures make certain undesirable outcomes inevitable. In such cases (spiralling debt is a classic example), a response of blaming the individual can be hugely discriminatory, whereas a holistic approach informed by the PCS analysis can be liberating and emancipatory.

Acknowledging and using our shared humanity

This is a skill that is rarely recognised and acknowledged in professional literature, but in many ways it is the supreme communication skill in ADP. It is far too easy to adopt the 'I'm the confident professional, the expert, and I know what is best for you' approach, while underneath we are often hurt, confused and unsure about ourselves at the personal level and in our own relationships. If we are honest, we are as susceptible to making a mess of things as anyone else, and often do just that. There is a skill, of course, in not allowing our own 'stuff' to get in the way of our professional relationships. To burden someone else with our problems, or to suggest in some superficial way that to share something of our own hurts will prove therapeutic to the other person, is widely recognised as being unhelpful, even dangerous. Our hurts may inform and even underpin our capacity to empathise with the other person, but they must stay firmly in the background.

There is nevertheless a subtle communication skill at work here. If we recognise and acknowledge our shared humanity with those we become involved with professionally, it will not only save us from the professional arrogance that distances us from people; more importantly, it will communicate to the other person that we too are human, vulnerable and at times hurting, as well as resilient, capable and open-hearted. If there is a tacit recognition that such capacities are open to us all, then we may be far more effective as 'wounded helpers' (Nouwen, 1999) than we realise.

## FINAL THOUGHTS

There has been a fascinating development to the discussion of ADP in the contemporary debate about spirituality. This is seen to be a far-reaching concept that includes religion, but also has far wider ramifications. Spirituality seeks to raise issues about meaning and purpose in people's lives, and to ask questions about the world view that people choose, consciously or unconsciously, in order to make sense of the world and their place within it. Some also argue for a social justice dimension to spirituality. Moss (2005: 71; and in Moss and Thompson, 2007), for example, argues that this concept of a person's world view, and the impact that a person's spirituality (S) has upon their lives in both positive and negative ways, is not only an important component of each level of the PCS analysis, it may even warrant its own additional 'dimension' (S for spiritual), thereby developing it into a PCSS analysis. For a recent critique of anti-oppressive practice, see Milner et al. (2015: 39–40).

## REFERENCES AND FURTHER READING

Holloway, M. and Moss, B. (2010) *Spirituality and Social Work*. Basingstoke: Palgrave Macmillan.

Milner, J., Myers, S. and O'Byrne, P. (2015) *Assessment in Social Work*, 4th edition. Basingstoke: Palgrave Macmillan.

Moss, B. (2005) *Religion and Spirituality*. Lyme Regis: Russell House.

Moss, B. and Thompson, N. (2007) 'Spirituality and equality', *Social and Public Policy Review*, 1 (1).

Nizra, V. and Williams, P. (2009) *Anti-Oppressive Practice in Health and Social Care.* London: Sage.

Nouwen, H. (1999) *The Wounded Healer: In Our Woundedness We Can Become a Source of Life for Others.* London: Darton, Longman and Todd.

Okitikpi, T. and Aymer, C. (2010) *Key Concepts in Anti-Discriminatory Social Work.* London: Sage.

Schön, D. (1983) *The Reflective Practitioner.* London: Temple Smith.

Schön, D. (1987) *Educating the Reflective Practitioner.* San Francisco, CA: Jossey Bass.

Thompson, N. (2011) *Effective Communication, A Guide for the People Professions*, 2nd edition. Basingstoke: Palgrave Macmillan.

Thompson, N. (2012) *The People Solutions Sourcebook*, 2nd edition. Basingstoke: Palgrave Macmillan.

Thompson, N. (2016) *Anti-Discriminatory Practice: Equality, Diversity and Social Justice*, 6th edition. Basingstoke: Palgrave Macmillan.

**RELATED CONCEPTS** acceptance; active listening; assessment; empathy; empowerment, resilience and a strengths perspective; feedback – giving and receiving; non-verbal communication; spirituality

**ENGAGING WITH THE PCF** context and organisations; diversity; rights and justice; values and ethics

**ENGAGING WITH THE NMC CODE** prioritise people; promote professionalism and trust

### Service user snippet

Josh (22), former drugs misuser:

'Don't speak to me about justice – I'm black and gay and proud of it … but people treat me like crap and that includes these so-called professionals. What do I have to do to be given respect, man?'

# ASSERTIVENESS

Working with other people is often a challenge. As people-workers, you are required to be good team players; to work within management guidelines; to contribute your ideas and insights; and to value the opinions, ideas and, at times, the specialist knowledge of others. And all the time you have to deal with the fascinating and, at times, bewildering and annoying character traits of those around you.

The challenge lies precisely in how you handle yourselves in this complex set of relationships. Perhaps you remember all too vividly occasions when you have tried tentatively to make a contribution to a discussion, only to feel 'slapped down' by another member of the group whose overpowering presence made you slink away with your tail between your legs, feeling undervalued and worthless. Such intimidating and overpowering behaviour not only makes you feel uncomfortable; it also saps your creative energies and diminishes your ability to make positive contributions. It also can make you fearful, and therefore the temptation to run away and take flight from the stressful encounter can be very strong.

There may also be occasions, however, when you feel so affronted, or even insulted, by another person's behaviour that your immediate *knee-jerk* reaction is to *give as good as you get*, and to respond with an angry riposte or a vitriolic tirade against the other person. 'No one speaks to me like that,' is your response, 'I'll show them what I'm made of'. And before you know it, a full-scale verbal boxing match has started, and no one wins.

## A NOTE OF CAUTION

There may be times when you are faced with an aggressive person who is threatening violence or who is making you feel too uncomfortable to continue. Your safety is paramount, so you need to remove yourself from any risk as soon as possible.

## Activity

Think about a situation at work or in your personal life where you have been on the receiving end of aggressive behaviour. Did you opt for fight or flight? How did this make you feel? What impact did this have upon your general wellbeing and your value as a team member? How would you have liked to have handled things differently?

*Handling things differently* takes us immediately into a discussion about assertiveness, which is an important skill and mindset for anyone involved in people-work. It involves being able to make your own contribution confidently whilst valuing and respecting the contribution made by others. Thompson (2012: 62–5) talks helpfully about a continuum of assertiveness, ranging at one end of the spectrum from being totally submissive and letting other people 'walk all over you', to the other extreme of being very aggressive, domineering, bullying even, stopping at nothing to ensure that you win the day at all costs. At each end of this continuum we will experience a degree of loss. If we allow ourselves to become 'doormats', we will lose a sense of self-worth, dignity and any thought that we have something useful to contribute. If we adopt an aggressive domineering approach, we will lose the respect and trust of those we are seeking to influence, and (if we are honest) have the feeling that we have let ourselves down by resorting to such insecure tactics that undermine the value base of our work.

Genuine assertiveness seeks to occupy the middle ground between these two extremes, and to foster a *win–win* mindset and value base. Each situation you encounter of course is different, and the contexts will vary. If you are in the midst of a particular crisis, perhaps dealing with someone who is critically ill, or needing to act quickly to protect a child or a vulnerable adult from abuse or harm, then proper lines of accountability will mean that, for the good of the person at risk, you need to act quickly, and to respond to orders and requests from the person in charge, whatever your personal views may be. Assertiveness is nevertheless essential if you are to value yourself, your colleagues and the unique contributions you all make to the organisations for which you work.

Assertiveness, therefore, is one example of your value base in action. It reflects the dignity and uniqueness of each and every person with whom you come into contact, and the value and worth you feel about yourself and the trust you have had placed in you by your employer. You have been entrusted to do a good job in partnership with other colleagues, both within your organisation and interprofessionally. You would be selling yourself short, as well as your colleagues and ultimately those for whom you care, if you do not maintain and develop skills of assertiveness in your day-to-day practice. You are not in the job to be liked: at times, you will need to fight hard on behalf of someone who is ill, vulnerable or in great need. They need you to stand up for them and to argue the case for them to the best of your ability, in a calm, professional but assertive way.

To achieve this, you need to be sensitive first of all to who you are, what your values are, and any potential 'baggage' you may carry with you in your interactions with other people. Your age, gender, experience and training; your position in the organisation; your race and culture are all important 'self-awareness' factors that contribute to this process. You may have had some personally difficult and painful experiences that colour and influence your ability to deal with similar situations with others. Some things might scare you, such as dying, bereavement, severe disability, domestic violence, AIDS, challenging people in authority, for example, and you might feel tempted to take flight when faced with these situations in other people's lives. To be assertive by being confident that you can face such personally challenging moments and deliver high standards of care to this person, or to represent them effectively, takes courage, but if you flinch then you are not delivering best practice. Similarly, you need to be sensitive to other people and how their behaviour can similarly be affected by such issues. If you can remain calm, and try *to hear the music behind the other person's words*, you are much more likely to achieve a win–win outcome. These are some of the essential skills of people-work that need to be practised and developed on a daily basis.

One of the most difficult areas for assertiveness is in challenging discriminatory and oppressive language and behaviour, both with the people you are trying to help and also at times with colleagues, especially if they are more senior to you within the organisation. Again, timing and context are important: on some occasions, it will feel right to say something immediately, by elegantly asking the person to stop using particular language or behaving in a certain way because you and your organisation find it unacceptable. On other occasions, however, it might be better to do this afterwards, either face to face or by sending a brief note or email. There will be instances, however, where the matter is sufficiently serious to make a complaint or to whistleblow; in such cases, however, it is wise to talk the issue through with a trusted colleague before you take action.

Assertiveness is not just a matter of what you say: it also involves *how* you say it and what message your non-verbal communication skills deliver to the other person. Effective assertiveness will involve a congruence between verbal and non-verbal communication and how you come across to the other person. We all instinctively sense when this does not happen; for example, when we ask a person if they are all right and they say 'Yes, I'm fine', but their general demeanour tells you they are far from all right. As people-workers, you need to ensure, therefore, that your non-verbal communication skills are enmeshed with the words you use so that you are communicating effectively and authentically.

---

### Group exercise

With the help of your tutor or supervisor, set up a multi-disciplinary discharge meeting to discharge an older adult back to his home. Roles could include an occupational therapist, physiotherapist, consultant, the older adult, his daughter/son and a (student) social worker or (student) nurse on placement. The student social worker's or nurse's assessment recommends the need for support services but at present there is no care in the community available. The consultant needs a hospital bed urgently and is adamant that this patient must be discharged today.

Decide in your respective roles what stance each of you wishes to take and then enact the role play to see what assertiveness skills are appropriate in this scenario.

After the role play has finished, discuss as a group what constitutes best practice. This group activity can be role-played several times with each group member taking it in turns to practise their assertiveness skills.

---

## FINAL THOUGHTS

Be encouraged! One of the spin-offs from developing your assertiveness skills is a greater sense of confidence in yourself and your professional abilities, and your effectiveness as a practitioner. Being genuinely assertive can lead to a win–win situation for yourself, those around you and the people whom you are seeking to help. But you will sometimes need support to achieve this, which is why it can be such a powerful issue to discuss in supervision.

## REFERENCES AND FURTHER READING

Hargie, O. (2016) *Skilled Interpersonal Communication*, 6th edition. Hove: Routledge.
McBride, P. (1998) *The Assertive Social Worker*. London: Routledge.
Thompson, N. (2011) *Effective Communication: A Guide for the People Professions*, 2nd edition. Basingstoke: Palgrave Macmillan.
Thompson, N. (2012) *The People Solutions Sourcebook*, 2nd edition. Basingstoke: Palgrave Macmillan.
Trevithick, P. (2012) *Social Work Skills and Knowledge: A Practice Handbook*, 3rd edition. Maidenhead: Open University.

**RELATED CONCEPTS** active listening; challenging; emotional intelligence (EI); feedback (giving and receiving); mediation skills; non-verbal communication; whistleblowing

**ENGAGING WITH THE PCF** context and organisation; skills and interventions; professional leadership; professionalism

**ENGAGING WITH THE NMC CODE** practise effectively; preserve safety

### Service user snippet

Justine (23), resident in a women's refuge:

'I got totally fed-up being treated like a doormat, but then my social worker helped me to stand up for myself and now I feel I am a new woman – wish I'd learned to do this ages ago.'

# ASSESSMENT

There can hardly be any aspect of people-work that does not involve the skill of assessment in one form or another. From the doctor making a complex diagnosis or the nurse keeping a careful eye on a patient's vital signs, to the solicitor trying to obtain a true picture of what happened when an offence took place; from the social worker having to make decisions about whether a child or a vulnerable adult needs to be safeguarded, to a manager of a care home having to decide whether someone is able to go into the town safely if unaccompanied: these are just some examples which illustrate the ways in which we can be called on to make assessments and judgements about other people.

At the less formal end of the spectrum, we all use some of these skills in our everyday life, when we make provisional assessments about another person's trustworthiness, for example. Of course, we sometimes get it wrong: we allow our prejudices and assumptions to cloud our judgement about the other person, but nevertheless we use assessment skills every day of our lives.

Within the professional context of people-work, however, assessment skills are of fundamental importance as they will frequently determine what level of service, if any, a person is entitled to receive. The evaluation of risk features strongly in this: we may be called upon to assess whether a person constitutes a risk to themselves or to others. We then need to devise responses that are not authoritarian or oppressive, but which work in partnership with the person involved. Taking an older person out of their home environment and placing them into residential care for their own protection when their various faculties are beginning to fail may be a wholly inappropriate response, for example. It may be far better to consider offering some support in their own home to enable them to stay in familiar surroundings with their pride and coping capacity intact.

The professional literature provides detailed discussions on assessment especially for social work (e.g. Trevithick, 2012: 174–84), and it is not appropriate to summarise all of the main issues here. It is useful, however, to draw attention to the very clear definition of assessment provided by Coulshed and Orme (2006: 24) who maintain that:

> Assessment is not a single event, it is an ongoing process, in which the client or service user participates, the purpose of which is to assist the social worker to understand people in relation to their environment. Assessment is also a basis for planning what needs to be done to maintain, improve or bring about change in the person or environment, or both.

This definition provides a salutary reminder that good assessment is a challenging activity which requires you to draw on a wide range of skills, knowledge and professional practice wisdom. It also takes place in the context where risk walks hand in hand with opportunity: you never really know what will work. So often skilled people-work involves what Munro (2011) calls *making decisions in conditions of uncertainty*, whereby you seek to balance the person's resilience and desire to control their own lives against the possibilities of harm, exploitation or abuse.

In identifying the communication skills inherent in all good assessment work, there are three skill sets which are of crucial importance. These may be summed up as: (1) helicopter vision; (2) partnership working; and (3) passing the 'abducted by aliens' test.

## HELICOPTER VISION

Social work is not alone in its commitment to holistic assessment: care for the whole person is a concept which pervades much nursing and medical practice, for example. The real challenge for any professional people-worker, however, is to take this holistic approach absolutely seriously, and to devise responses to individual problems and situations that take into account the wider contexts in which people live their lives. This is what Thompson (2012: 119ff) means by 'helicopter vision': it is the determination to gain as detailed and as comprehensive an overview as possible of the 'person in context'. This means, therefore, that we do not just focus on the physical, emotional, psychological and spiritual aspects of a person's individual life, but also explore the social, cultural and societal dimensions which may impact upon their immediate difficulties. For example, the impact of poverty, racism, disablism, the 'debt culture' or homophobia on a person's life may be of huge importance, and any solution that does not take into account these factors is bound to be short-lived.

In terms of communication skills, therefore, an effective assessment will attempt to explore these wider issues and their impact upon the person. This approach also counteracts the pathologising tendency among some welfare professionals to assume that a person's problems are all their fault (sometimes referred to as the 'deficit model'), whereas the reality is often that the person has been struggling valiantly against massive societal pressures. To be able to appreciate these wider dimensions to a person's difficulties can be a significant aspect of empathic attunement, and can re-energise them to explore structural as well as individual solutions.

### Group exercise

With the help of your tutor or supervisor, choose a scenario from your own practice setting. Then practise using the 'helicopter vision' by asking as many open questions as possible only regarding that person (see if you can ask 21 of them!). You may not know the answers of course, but the questions are important. What are the wider societal and cultural factors that may exacerbate the person's difficulties? How does an appreciation of these wider issues help you come to a richer assessment of what this person really needs?

# PARTNERSHIP WORKING

Partnership working is a theme that pervades all social work practice, but is important in many other aspects of people-work. For it to be more than a 'practice mantra', however, it requires you to develop and practise a range of communication skills which, at all levels, give the clear signal to the other person that partnership working really is 'the name of the game'.

It is temptingly easy for professional workers not only to feel that 'they know best', but also to convey this to the person they are working with. From this, there flows a subtle movement towards dependency, where the professional 'takes over' with the tacit message 'trust me, I am a professional – do what I tell you and all will be well'. Many people, feeling vulnerable and unsure of how best to proceed, fall gratefully into this trap, only to discover further down the line that they have been short-changed by having their resilience, their expertise, their capacity to change and to take responsibility for their lives, called into serious question. Maybe the professional worker did not intend this to happen; but by not practising the skills of partnership working this was the outcome.

It may be the case, of course, that in the early days of the professional relationship, the other person needs you to take some action on their behalf. A threat of immediate eviction, for example, is usually best removed, or at least delayed, by appropriate professional intervention. But if this is all that is done, and the person then walks away with a sigh of relief, they will soon discover that the 'evil day' returns once more to haunt them. As a people-worker, you need to establish a trusting relationship where the real issues and problems are identified, and a clear strategy is devised, to help the person deal with them.

You can then begin to suggest to people that they are the experts in their own lives; that they know what is best for them and their family; that they know what needs to be done. If you can begin to articulate these values, then your role as a professional will be to encourage, to support, to provide information and to work with them to help them effect the changes that will be necessary if they are to emerge from their current cluster of problems. If you do all the work, and the person in difficulty remains a grateful but passive spectator, the chances are that whatever caused the problems will recur.

The skill in this approach is not just in the words and gestures that you use, but in your essential value base, to ensure that respect and dignity are accorded to the other person in every possible way.

## Activity

Put yourself in the position of going to someone for help with a difficult problem. How would you like to be treated? What would partnership working mean for you? How would you feel if you were not treated in this way?

A further crucial dimension to partnership working is interprofessional collaboration. The history of people-work is littered with examples and reports where communication between relevant professionals has broken down or has not even been considered, resulting in abuse and neglect going unnoticed, unreported or inadequately tackled. One key question you always need to ask, therefore, in making your assessments is this: what other agencies/professionals are (or need to be) involved here, and what role must I play in facilitating this?

## PASSING THE 'ABDUCTED BY ALIENS' TEST

This somewhat tongue-in-cheek, light-hearted title refers to the importance of accurate accessible recording. Parker (2010: 136) uses this idea to capture an important issue, which he describes as follows:

> If you were abducted by aliens tomorrow, would someone else in the office or agency be able to pick up your work and understand it?

The implications for assessment are clear. No matter how well you have worked in partnership with your service user, if this is not fully, accurately and clearly recorded there is a chance that all will be lost. Professional people-workers often lament the bureaucracy of paperwork and endless reports, but in truth they are the mechanisms for recording important work and for ensuring that others have access to it. Records and reports are also often essential before decisions can be taken by managers to allocate resources.

This means that you need to record all relevant information clearly, succinctly and in plain English, and to state clearly where decisions need to be taken. Recommendations should also be clearly indicated. Most agencies, of course, have standard documents and pro formas for recording information, and it is important that these are used properly. With multi-agency working becoming increasingly important, the need for accurate recording is paramount.

One further aspect of this is the right of access to information that service users, carers, patients and clients now have to their records. You need to have clear in your own mind your agency policy concerning access to records, and to make sure that you consider this when completing your reports. It is best practice to share assessment documents with your service user, and for them to sign them and to have copies, although you will first need to check your agency policy.

## THE COMMON ASSESSMENT FRAMEWORK (CAF)

One further aspect of assessment concerns working with children and families. In 2000, the Department of Health produced its *Framework for the Assessment of Children in Need and their Families*. This is required reading for anyone working with children and families in a professional context. The report states clearly that:

Assessing whether a child is in need and the nature of these needs requires a systematic approach which uses the same framework or conceptual map for gathering and analysing information about all children and their families, but discriminates effectively between different types and levels of need ... It requires a thorough understanding of the developmental needs of children; the capacities of parents or caregivers to respond appropriately to those needs, and the impact of wider family and environmental factors on parenting capacity and children. (CWDC, 2000: 17)

In exploring these issues, the report produced its assessment framework triangle, which indicates the range of issues that need to be taken into account in safeguarding and promoting the welfare of a child. The three arms of the triangle are: (1) the child's developmental needs; (2) parenting capacity; and (3) family and environmental factors. It is only when all of these factors have been taken into account that a holistic assessment can be made. In this respect, the framework reflects the key skills and issues we have highlighted in this discussion, and underlines their importance for the assessment process.

The Common Assessment Framework (CAF) builds on this work by offering a standardised approach to conducting an assessment to help in the early identification of a child's additional needs, and to facilitate a coordinated response to ensure these needs are met. This often involves some Team Around the Child (TAC) interprofessional meetings with the key agencies working with the child and the family. The seminal report from Munro (2011) into child protection procedures is essential reading to help you understand and practise high-quality assessments with children and their families.

## Group exercise

With the help of your tutor or supervisor, obtain a copy of the Common Assessment Framework and look carefully at the assessment triangle with its various components. Chapter 2 provides a detailed discussion of what is involved, and deserves careful study.

1   Examine some core CAF documentation, and evaluate its effectiveness as an assessment tool.
2   Now find some assessment documentation used in connection with safeguarding adults (the Care Quality Commission has a lot of resources available on their website www.cqc.org.uk). Compare and contrast these with the CAF approach.

As will be clear from the tasks in the Group Exercise above, it is important to emphasise that there are some important issues being raised here in connection with adult care. The Care Act 2014, for example, emphasises the importance of personalisation where people take increasing responsibility for their own care and wellbeing, and how they prefer resources to be most effectively used. This approach, together with the emphasis upon the needs of carers, has highlighted the shared, partnership aspect of assessment. The service user is being empowered far more to 'call the shots' by the worker who is *sitting beside* rather than *standing above*.

## Mental capacity

One so far unacknowledged strand running through our discussion concerns mental capacity. For everyone, decision making is a feature of everyday life, consciously or unconsciously, sometimes spontaneously, sometimes after a lengthy period of thought. Capacity to make decisions is therefore an important aspect of the assessment process; if someone is unable for whatever reason to come to an informed decision, then this must be taken seriously, with reasons being clearly stated.

Having mental capacity to make decisions means that a person will be able to:

- understand all the information needed to make a decision;
- use or think about the information;
- remember the information; and
- be able to communicate their decision to someone else. (www.rethink.org)

The Mental Capacity Act 2005 is an important 'tool' therefore in helping you understand and work with this issue if someone has an impairment or disturbance in their functioning of the mind or brain.

You also need to be aware that some people can experience a fluctuating capacity. For example, they may have a condition which affects their capacity (e.g. a urinary tract infection) but when treated, their capacity returns. The Mental Capacity Act 2005 has now been applied by courts to a range of decision-making scenarios including consent to medical treatment and to sexual relationships.

## FINAL THOUGHTS

Good assessment skills are at the heart of all people-work. You owe it to yourself, your agency and crucially the people with whom you work to ensure that you are developing your ability to work in this complex, ambiguous and at times uncertain territory.

## REFERENCES AND FURTHER READING

Children's Workforce Development Council (CWDC) (2000) *Common Assessment Framework*. Leeds: CWDC.
Coulshed, V. and Orme, J. (2006) *Social Work Practice: An Introduction*, 4th edition. Basingstoke: Macmillan/BASW.
Department of Health (DH) (2000) *Framework for the Assessment of Children in Need and their Families*. London: DH.
Department of Health (DH) (2014) *Care Act 2014*. London: DH.

Gardner, A. (2014) *Personalisation and Social Work*, 2nd edition. Exeter: Learning Matters.

Hopkins, G. (1998) *Plain English for Social Services: A Guide to Better Communication*. Lyme Regis: Russell House.

Martin, R. (2010) *Social Work Assessment*. Exeter: Learning Matters.

Milner, J., Myers, S. and O'Byrne, P. (2015) *Assessment in Social Work*, 4th edition. Basingstoke: Palgrave Macmillan.

Munro, E. (2011) *The Munro Review of Child Protection: Final Report – a Child-centred System (cm 8062)*. Norwich: TSO.

O'Rourke, L. (2010) *Recording in Social Work: Not Just an Administrative Task*. Bristol: Policy Press.

Parker, J. (2010) *Effective Practice Learning in Social Work*, 2nd edition. Exeter: Learning Matters.

Thompson, N. (2012) *The People Solutions Sourcebook*. Basingstoke: Palgrave Macmillan.

Trevithick, P. (2012) *Social Work Skills: A Practice Handbook*, 3rd edition. Maidenhead: Open University Press.

Wallace, C. and Davies, M. (2009) *Sharing Assessment in Health and Social Care: A Practical Handbook for Interprofessional Working*. London: Sage.

Woodcock Ross, J. (2016) *Specialist Communication Skills for Social Workers: Developing Professional Capability*, 2nd edition. Basingstoke: Palgrave Macmillan.

 Web resources

Rethink Mental Illness – www.rethink.org (accessed 11/09/2019)

NICE guidelines, 'Decision-making and mental capacity' – www.nice.org.uk/NG108 (accessed 15/10/19)

Social Care Institute for Excellence, MCA Directory – www.scie.org.uk/mca-directory (accessed 15/10/19)

Assess Right, MCA website – www.assessright.co.uk (accessed 15/10/19)

**RELATED CONCEPTS** empathy; establishing a professional relationship; interprofessional collaboration

**ENGAGING WITH THE PCF** all domains are relevant to this theme

**ENGAGING WITH THE NMC CODE** prioritise people; preserve safety

Service user snippet

Jasvinder (15), after a youth justice court appearance:

'I hated every minute of it … it was like being put on trial … ugh!'

# BARRIERS TO GOOD COMMUNICATION

A barrier to good communication is any action, behaviour, attitude, world view or physical arrangement (such as room layout) that discourages the other person from feeling comfortable, accepted and valued, thereby reducing your, and their, ability to communicate positively and effectively. This topic involves active listening skills, how you put your values into practice, how you deal with non-verbal communication, all of which are discussed elsewhere in this book. For the moment it is important to recognise and deal with some of the physical barriers to good communication.

There are some situations, of course, where physical barriers are both sensible and necessary for the protection of the worker. There are classic examples of this within the prison service and of how arrangements can be made for the safety of visitors. But many reception areas for public services have, from time to time, employed security screens in the hope of discouraging violence or abusive behaviour and for the protection of staff. These have not always worked, however, and have sometimes given the message that violent behaviour is being expected. Some people find such screens to be so impersonal that they provoke a suspicious, even aggressive, response. They much prefer to create an open, warm and human environment that respects the individual and encourages them in turn to behave respectfully towards the worker. It is also possible that screens can put confidentiality at risk if people feel that they have to speak more loudly in order to make themselves heard. Screens in GP surgeries are good examples of this.

## Activity

Think of some situations and settings you know where there are security screens or similar barriers in operation. Do you think they are effective? Make a list of the advantages and disadvantages. In what settings might screens be essential?

As people-workers, you need to give careful thought to how furniture is arranged within the rooms and spaces where you meet with people and interview them. You need to give due attention to what seems open, welcoming and conducive to good shared communication, but not to overlook health and safety risk factors. These will include ensuring that:

**B**

- You can leave the room easily and quickly in case of difficulty.
- Panic buttons are visible and accessible but not 'in your face'.
- Decorative objects are not easily available to use as weapons or missiles.

Room layout communicates something to those who use the room, both in being welcome and open, but also in reinforcing boundaries for behaviour that is deemed unacceptable and that might put people at risk. Posters about behaviour, and the type of actions and language that are not acceptable, are also further examples of the ways in which boundaries can be clearly established.

The way in which professional workers, including doctors and solicitors, arrange their offices is also instructive. Do they sit behind a desk to enhance their status and power? Or do they sit beside it so that they are more accessible to people who come to see them?

All of the above are examples of a broad understanding of what barrier gestures involve, sometimes in emphasising or minimising the power differential between professionals and those who use their services, and sometimes in establishing the boundaries of what is acceptable conduct. The message is clear: go beyond this barrier and you could be in trouble.

## NON-VERBAL BARRIER GESTURES

More generally, however, within a wide range of people-work activities, barrier gestures are deemed to be unhelpful and discouraging to good communication. Sometimes these are very significant and obvious; other examples may seem more trivial and irritating. The overall impact of a barrier gesture upon the other person, however, is the message that we are not paying full attention to them, or even that we do not really want to hear what they have to say.

Some examples of barrier gestures which workers have been known to use, consciously or unconsciously, and the impact these can have, include:

- sitting with arms firmly crossed over the chest = a very defensive 'don't come near me' approach;
- sitting slumped in the chair = I'm too 'chilled out' to be bothered with you;
- fiddling with a book, pen or other object = this is a really interesting object I have got here. I prefer playing with this to listening to you;
- jangling your keys and change in your pocket = I'll be glad to get away from here into my car or to do some serious shopping;
- fiddling with your hair, ears or face = I'm feeling rather uneasy with this conversation and need to engage in some self-comforting activity;
- gazing out of the window = there are far more interesting things happening out there than in this interview;
- glancing at your watch surreptitiously = I'll be glad when this interview is over;
- answering phone calls during the interview = this person is not important enough for me to give them uninterrupted time – see how busy and important I am though;

- placing yourself behind the desk = now, little person, what can I do for you today – see how important I am and how lucky you are to have me to talk to.

The interpretations given to each of these barrier gestures are perhaps tongue-in-cheek and slightly exaggerated, but they make a serious point. There are a number of things you can do during an interview that can be off-putting to the other person, and give a message that you are not really interested in what they have to say. Some barrier gestures you can perhaps easily identify and rectify, but everyone has their idiosyncrasies that they are hardly aware of. These include the little mannerisms, which in themselves really do not matter much and may in some situations be rather endearing, but which in a professional interview could be irritating and off-putting. The only way of spotting these, of course, is either to ask permission for a trusted colleague to sit in with you and give you feedback, or in a training context to video yourself in an interview, and watch yourself afterwards in action.

The reason for stressing this is not to make you so self-conscious that you become wooden, unnatural and awkward – exactly the opposite. It is to help you focus totally, warmly and openly on the other person, and to remove anything which distracts from enabling them to feel they have been fully listened to and accepted.

## READING THE SIGNS

This awareness, of course, will help you to deal with barrier gestures that service users, clients or patients use when being interviewed by you. In the discussion about non-verbal communication, it is argued that all of us communicate non-verbally all the time through our body language. Just as you need as people-workers to be aware of what you are communicating to your service users through *your* body language, so too can you learn to 'read the signs' from other people's body language, in order to appreciate what they are trying to say to you without necessarily being able to put it into words.

---

### Group exercise

With the help of your tutor or supervisor, discuss the incident where a male doctor was reported to the General Medical Council (GMC) for asking a Muslim woman to remove her veil so he could hear (and see) what she was saying.

Are there any circumstances where the removal of a niqab or burka is necessary for good communication? If so, what would best practice in such circumstances involve?

---

The communication skills needed here are your ability to read the signs accurately, and to respond in ways that help to draw the other person into the interview, and not drive a deeper wedge between you. It is helpful, therefore, to be able to put into words what you suspect the barrier gestures are communicating to you. For example:

'J, I can see from how you are sitting that you don't really want to be here.'

'I guess, J, that if I were in your shoes, I would want to be somewhere else right now.'

'Tell me if I have got it wrong, J, but you seem pretty angry and fed up to me.'

'Feeling bored, J?'

'J, how can I help you get a bit more out of our time together today?'

Sometimes, however, we can misunderstand other people's gestures. For example, in some cultures, it is a sign of respect to someone in authority not to maintain eye contact with them. If this were to be misinterpreted as being disrespectful, a serious breakdown in communication could well follow.

## MIRRORING

One of the skills which sometimes works to help unlock someone's barrier gestures is called 'mirroring'. Stated simply, this approach suggests that, as the worker, you mirror the gestures that the other person is using: for example, if they are sitting with arms firmly crossed, you do the same for a while. And then, as you talk to them, slowly begin to unfold your arms. You may find that they start to copy your actions and begin to visibly relax. It is worth an occasional try, but it needs to be done subtly, and there is no guarantee that it will work.

## TRICKY MOMENTS

There will be occasions when there can be no doubt what the person is feeling. You may be faced with someone who raises a hand or shakes a fist at you, or who suddenly stands over you in a threatening manner. Your personal safety may well then be at risk, and you will need to decide how best to respond. Initially, try to defuse the situation by saying something like:

'J, I know you are angry and upset, but please stop doing that.'

'J, please sit down – it does not help either of us if you try to threaten me.'

'J, I can't help you if you treat me like this.'

'J, violence doesn't solve anything – it really doesn't – please sit down.'

If the situation escalates, then the time for talking is over, and you need to leave the room as quickly as possible and summon help. Your safety is paramount.

## FINAL THOUGHTS

There are, of course, no guarantees that you will break through the barriers that are being erected, but at least if you can begin to put into words what you suspect the person is feeling, it will go some way towards helping them realise that they are being listened to and respected.

## REFERENCES AND FURTHER READING

Ellis, R.B., Gates, B. and Kenworthy, N. (2003) *Interpersonal Communication in Nursing: Theory and Practice*, 2nd edition. Edinburgh: Churchill Livingstone.
Thompson, N. (2011) *Effective Communication: A Guide for the People Professions*, 2nd edition. Basingstoke: Palgrave Macmillan.
Trevithick, P. (2012) *Social Work Skills: A Practice Handbook*, 3rd edition. Maidenhead: Open University Press.
Woodcock Ross, J. (2016) *Specialist Communication Skills for Social Workers: Developing Professional Capability*, 2nd edition. Basingstoke: Palgrave Macmillan.

**RELATED CONCEPTS** anti-discriminatory practice; empathy; non-verbal communication

**ENGAGING WITH THE PCF** skills and interventions; professionalism

**ENGAGING WITH THE NMC CODE** practise effectively; promote professionalism and trust

Service user snippet

Jane (15):

'I couldn't believe it – she kept looking at her watch thinking I wouldn't notice. It really put me off. Well, two can play at that game. I can tell you!'

# BREAKING BAD NEWS

If there is one thing arguably more difficult than receiving bad news, it is having to break bad news to someone. If you have ever had to do this, you will know how distressing it can be for the 'breaker' and the receiver. Your stomach churns as the moment approaches; you worry about how the person will react; you wonder how it would be if the situation were in reverse; and perhaps memories of bad news you have received in the past come flooding back. Without doubt, this is not territory you would choose to be in.

But sometimes, as part of your job as people-workers, you are called upon to undertake this important but painful task. And while there are no easy golden rules to guarantee that such occasions will go well, some guidelines to help you are set out below.

First of all, it is helpful to explore some of the situations where, as a professional, you may be called on to break bad news. There are occasions when you may have to tell someone that:

- you are taking their child into care;
- their relative has died;
- they have a terminal illness;
- they are being made redundant;
- their teenage son has been arrested;
- they cannot receive the services they had hoped for.

As a nurse you may well be called upon to sit with someone who has just been told of a life-limiting illness, or has just lost a close relative.

## Activity

1   The list above provides just a few examples. Spend a few moments adding to it, both from your own experience in your work setting, and from likely scenarios that you know other colleagues have had to deal with.
2   Look again at your list. Try to identify what it is that worries you most about having to break bad news. Jot your thoughts down before you move on to the next section of this discussion.

You have now set the scene for exploring this difficult aspect of communication skills. The section that follows outlines a way of approaching such situations in an appropriate professional manner, which puts the other person's needs 'in the driving seat', but also helps you best prepare. The news you are about to break will come as a shock; you cannot disguise that, nor minimise the impact it might have. What you can do, however, is to remember that, if you do your best and follow the guidelines we suggest, you will earn the gratitude of that person (in due course, if not straightaway) for the way you have handled it. How you deal with this situation *will* make a difference to the person receiving the news.

## PREPARATION

Although you may not know the person to whom you are going to break bad news well enough to predict how they will respond – they may get very distressed or 'go into their shell' in a protective silence, for example – you should know yourself well enough to realise that good preparation is essential both at the 'head level' and at the 'heart level'.

### Head-level preparation

'Head-level' preparation is about being as sure as you can be concerning the information you are going to be asked about, once you have broken the bad news. Try to put yourself into the other person's shoes and anticipate what their questions might be; find out in advance as much information as you can. This will involve being very clear about what you do know and can find out about, and what questions will have to remain unanswered. For example, if you are breaking news about a person involved in an accident, or who has a serious medical condition, it is likely that there will be many things you do not know about, and which may be beyond your professional expertise anyway. In such situations, you must be honest and say you do not know; but you may be able to refer them to other colleagues who will be able to provide these important answers.

There is another set of difficult questions, however, that no one will ever be able to answer fully, and these are the big 'why?' questions that people often ask in moments of profound shock. Frequently, these questions pose deep existential concerns for that person's world view, which may be on the brink of disintegration in the face of such bad news. For example:

- Why did God allow this to happen?
- Why did God take this person away and leave me?
- What have I done to deserve this?
- Why did it happen to him/her – he/she was such a lovely person?

These and many other searching questions brook no easy answer, but, nevertheless, can place the breaker of bad news in a difficult situation. It is worth some prior thought, therefore, to prepare yourself for responding to such painful, challenging moments. This is important whether or not you yourself belong to a faith community or believe in God, Allah or a Supreme Being. It is tempting sometimes, for example, to offer someone in distress an insight into your own world view in the hope that it will comfort them in their moment of anguish. A devout Christian or Muslim, for instance, may believe that whatever happens must somehow be the will and purpose of God or Allah. 'Insha'Allah' is how Muslims would express this: it is God's will. By definition, there can be nothing that happens that falls outside the will and purpose of the Divine Being. But to state this to a person who has no such belief could alienate them from you at the very moment when you have the opportunity as another human being to be open and supportive to them. By contrast, the person who has received the bad news may have a faith which can accommodate this disaster, and tells you so, but you may feel appalled by this world view to which you would feel totally unable to subscribe yourself. Then there are searching questions for people who belong to a faith community but whose belief in God is shattered by the awful news they have just received. They may ask you how they will be able to cope from now on.

The variations are endless, but in many ways the issue for you is the same. Whatever your own world view is; whether or not you subscribe to a religious faith; no matter how painful or upsetting you may find the scenario to be personally, your principal responsibility is to the person who has just received the news you have brought to them. It is not for you to bring your own 'agenda' into play with how you do, or do not, view the world, and whether you do or do not have a religious faith. Your task is to be as open as possible to the hurt, the anguish and the confusion that the person is experiencing. Easy answers are a misnomer: they are not answers, and they are usually offered to make *you* feel better, not the person you are working with.

The most helpful responses, therefore, will be the ones that treat the other person with the utmost seriousness and respect; that listen to their pain and distress and do not seek to offer trite statements, however well-intentioned; and which seek to 'hear the music beyond the words' when such questions are posed. In other words, if you can respond to, and acknowledge, the pain and confusion that these questions represent, you may be far more helpful because the person begins to feel that you really are listening to them, and have begun to realise the depth of their loss.

## Heart-level preparation

These issues have already brought us into the second aspect of preparation, the 'heart-level' or emotional preparation. It is important that any disquiet, nervousness or even fear at having to undertake such a task as breaking bad news does not get in the way. Nor must you allow your own distress or upset to intrude into the interview or meeting that you are about to conduct. In other words, you need to take your emotional temperature, and talk through with someone you can trust how you are feeling about this task. Far better to do your crying as part of your own preparation than let your own emotions spill over into the interview when you are having to deal with the tears of the other person. But even if it is not likely to reduce you to tears, it is still important to talk through with someone else how you are going to handle the situation, what words you are going to use to break the bad news and how you will seek to respond to some of the issues that will inevitably arise.

This is not to say that everything will go as you have planned – far from it – but you will be surprised how much better you will handle the encounter if you have taken the trouble to do some of this important preparation in advance.

One further tip: it is useful to jot down some key information to leave with the person you are going to see. The chances are that they will be in shock and will not remember details very well. If you have left information for them in writing, including some contact details for yourself or others, that will be a great help. But you will need to give careful thought to what you write down.

## PLANNING FOR THE MEETING

Much of what follows is based on a protocol for breaking bad news developed to help medical professionals in their roles, but it is relevant and easily adaptable to other people-work contexts. The SPIKES protocol – setting, perception, invitation, knowledge, emotions, strategy/summary – was originally developed by Baile and Buckman (2000), and you will find it helpful to consider the issues they raise when you are involved in breaking bad news yourself.

### S: the setting

Where the interview or meeting takes place clearly makes a big difference. If it is to be in your own office, you will have far more control over what happens. You will be able to ensure a private uninterrupted space, where the phone is on 'divert' and staff know you are not to be interrupted.

You will be able to ensure that a box of tissues and refreshments are available, and that the layout of the room is appropriate. But you may also need to take into account whether the person will be able to return home safely or whether they will need someone to be with them for support while they are in a state of shock.

You may find, however, that you have to conduct this discussion in a less favourable setting. You may have to break bad news to someone on a hospital ward, or in a day or residential setting; or when visiting someone in prison where you have far less control over the environment you will be working in. It is important, therefore, to do everything in your power to seek a private room in which to conduct the interview. Contact the staff in advance; explain that you have some sensitive issues to explore, and that you will need privacy. This will be especially important if the person has hearing difficulties: you will not want to have to raise your voice to impart such difficult news. But if privacy cannot be guaranteed, you will need to think about how to position yourself so that you can speak in as quiet a voice as possible during the interview.

If you are breaking bad news in someone's home, there are other considerations to bear in mind. One distinct advantage is that the person will be on home territory, and will not have to make the journey back from your office to their home after hearing the news. But home territory brings other hazards. Music, pets, television, other people being present, children, casual callers, phone calls: all of these can impact upon the meeting you are trying to conduct. Again, you will need to introduce the reason for your visit early on, and, if need be, invite the person to prepare themselves appropriately. You may need to ask for the TV to be turned off. It is not your territory, but do try to take some control so that you have a reasonable chance of doing your difficult job effectively.

Sometimes the setting will be a telephone call, and this too needs careful thought. You will be surprised perhaps by the sheer volume of information that your tone of voice can convey over the phone. If you do not believe that, then think about occasions when you have been expecting news (good or bad) to be conveyed to you by telephone. The chances are that you will sense the outcome of the phone call in the first few seconds, simply by the tone of voice of the person making the call, and how they go about the task of talking to you. If you are using the phone to make an urgent appointment to visit someone to break bad news face to face, you will need to decide how much to say to them in advance. If you make it sound too light-hearted, they will not be at all prepared for what you have to say; if you do manage to convey the seriousness of the situation, you may find yourself giving most, if not all, of the information in that phone call, especially as they will inevitably ask you questions about why you want to pay them a visit. Here again, preparation about what you will say and how you will say it are invaluable. If you do have to tell them the news over the phone, you will need to ask them if they have anyone with them or whether they are sitting down, because you have some bad news for them.

Finally, you may find that, as is often the case with the police, you are having to 'cold call'. Unlike the police, however, where the unexpected visit from uniformed officers immediately conveys some important information, this may not be the case with you. Again, you need to be prepared, with a form of words to use which deals sensitively but clearly with the reason for your visit. Also, you must ensure that you have your ID card or badge with you so that they know they are receiving a visit from a bona fide worker.

## P: the other person's perceptions

You will have had time to rehearse what you need to say and how you are going to handle the meeting. But for the person on the receiving end, this could be a bolt out of the blue for which they are completely unprepared. In such situations, it is likely that they will not take in the news you are giving to them. It is important, therefore, that you try to assess the person's perceptions, and how they seem to be absorbing and understanding what you are seeking to convey. Their reaction may suggest that they have not fully appreciated the seriousness of what you are telling them. It is helpful, therefore, to go over the ground as many times as is necessary, if need be by asking them to 'play back' to you the key features so that you know they have taken it in. As mentioned in the section on preparation, it is useful to have some key information available to give to them in writing, as they may be in shock for a while and unable to take in fully what you are saying.

## I: invitation

Another issue to bear in mind is that all professionals have their own jargon which they use as easily and at times as unthinkingly as drawing breath. With the best will in the world and with every intention to communicate clearly, you may still sometimes fail to guard against this when talking to people. This means that you must be prepared to go over the ground more than once, and to invite them to ask questions if they feel they have not fully understood some of the terms you have used. 'There is no such thing as a silly question' is a very useful golden rule to share with them.

Sometimes, of course, further information is not always appropriate. The person may feel they have got enough to deal with and do not want to know any more, at least as far as the immediate moment is concerned. In medical contexts, there is often the issue of the extent to which people understand the full implications of a medical diagnosis, but other professionals have similar situations to deal with, where people may not always fully appreciate the implications of what is being told to them. It is important, therefore, to leave the invitation open; to invite people to think about what has been said, and to jot down any issues that they may wish to ask you about next time you meet.

## K: knowledge

How you convey information to the person is important; the timing of it and how you control the flow of information can make all the difference between a successful and unsuccessful interview. As an example of this, think about meeting with an insurance sales representative, or a double-glazing salesperson. How often have such interviews led to the potential buyer feeling bamboozled and totally confused by information overload? They reach a point where they find it impossible even to ask a sensible question, and just long for the meeting to end so that they can catch their breath. This is the worst possible scenario for you to emulate when breaking bad news.

It is important, therefore, to convey information in bite-sized chunks that the person can understand, and which you can easily check off as the interview unfolds. This is a major communication skill because it requires you to be aware of how the person is absorbing information. You want to avoid going too slowly, which can feel patronising, or too swiftly, which can feel insensitive. Finding the 'middle way' is the key to a successful interview, and this will be different for each person you work with. The main point always to bear in mind, therefore, is that the imparting of information is only half the story: how it is received and understood is the other half, and if you do not take responsibility for checking this other half of the equation, you will not have done your job at all well.

## E: explore emotions and empathise

How someone receives the information you are giving them will often be indicated and measured by their emotional response. It is important, therefore, that you have

**B**

prepared yourself to deal with this aspect of the interview in a sensitive way. Sometimes the immediate bursting into tears is easier to deal with than someone going into an impenetrable silence. But even tears can be challenging, especially if there are gender issues involved. Not all men find it easy to cry; some more readily express an angry response. Some people find it difficult to be with men who are able to cry; occasionally it stimulates upset or distress within us. The skill of saying nothing while the person expresses their tearfulness or anger should not be underestimated. It is sometimes helpful simply to acknowledge to them that you realise how painful this is for them, and that you are not trying to rush them through such an emotional response to the news you have broken. Just saying to them that you realise this news will inevitably have been deeply upsetting and disturbing will be a small step towards achieving a degree of empathy with them. And to have someone perceptive and sensitive enough to stay with them during these emotional moments can make all the difference to how they deal with things subsequently.

## S: strategy and summary

Interviews need to come to an end, and how this type of interview concludes is very much up to your skill and judgement, and how much time you have allowed for the meeting. There is always the chance, of course, that in a person's home the end of the interview may be precipitated by a child bursting into the room, or the dog creating a diversion, or the phone ringing. But even so, you will want to ensure that the meeting closes in as caring and planned a way as possible. You do not want to be walking away when the person is still deeply distressed.

You need to have a strategy, therefore, for dealing with what needs to happen next. This may involve contacting other professionals; arranging a further meeting; fixing a time when you will ring them to see how they are. In extreme cases, you may need to contact medical services to arrange for an assessment or other medical intervention. It is always useful to offer a brief, sensitive summary of the story so far, and what you have agreed to do next, and to leave information in writing, especially any important contact details.

---

### Group exercise

With the help of your tutor or supervisor, identify some scenarios from your work settings, real or imagined, where bad news would be involved, and use the SPIKES model to explore how you would undertake that task.

---

## FINAL THOUGHTS

As we indicated at the outset, there are so many different scenarios for breaking bad news that it is impossible to think about, let alone plan for, every eventuality. What can be said, however, is that in breaking bad news, it will be your approach, your values and your personality as a worker that will shine through clearest of all. If you develop the skills to do it well, you will earn the gratitude of those you work with more than you will perhaps ever realise.

There can be no denying that such work is stressful and at times upsetting. It is no disgrace to feel emotionally drained after such an encounter, or to find that you have suddenly become 'weepy' afterwards. It is crucial, therefore, to take good care of yourself, personally and professionally, by finding an appropriate person to talk to afterwards, to offload and to get back into shape emotionally to work with other people.

## REFERENCES AND FURTHER READING

Baile, W.F. and Buckman, R. (2000) 'SPIKES: a six step protocol for delivering bad news', *The Oncologist*, 5 (4): 302–11.
Buckman, R. (2000) *I Don't Know What to Say*, 2nd edition. London: Pan Books.
Buckman, R. and Kason, Y. (1992) *How to Break Bad News: A Guide for Health Care Professionals*. Baltimore, MD: Johns Hopkins University Press.

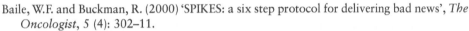

**RELATED CONCEPTS** active listening; dealing with upset service users; empathy; non-verbal communication; religion; spirituality; supervision

**ENGAGING WITH THE PCF** skills and interventions; values and ethics

**ENGAGING WITH THE NMC CODE** prioritise people

---

### Service user snippet

Alison (45):

'It was the worst day of my life. My beautiful Annabel had been rushed into hospital all of a sudden … and after what seemed like hours of waiting the surgeon and a nurse came out to tell me what had happened. I could see from their faces before a word was spoken that I had lost my precious daughter. After the surgeon left, the nurse stayed behind. She was so kind – she stayed with me – held my hand … explained everything – she made such a difference … I can't thank her enough.'

# CHAIRING MEETINGS

An increasingly important communication skill for anyone involved with people-work is that of chairing meetings. Meetings themselves are channels of communication, both for those physically present and participating in the discussion and decision making, and also for those not attending who may need to discover what was decided by accessing the minutes.

Whether the meetings are fairly low-key, or of huge significance – such as a case conference – some of the principles and issues are the same when it comes to the task of chairing them successfully.

## Activity

Next time you attend a formal meeting, spend some time trying to identify how well the meeting is being chaired. What seems to make it go well (or not)? What does the chair do, or not do? How involved do the participants seem to be? Are there any frustrating aspects of the meeting? If so, what are they? How would you handle it differently?

## GUIDELINES AND PRINCIPLES

In fact, chairing a meeting is not all that difficult if you keep certain guidelines and principles firmly in mind. One of the most important of these is preparation.

### Preparation

There are some basic points to remember before any meeting takes place. These include:

- Why is the meeting necessary? What purpose(s) will it fulfil?
- Who needs to be present in order for the meeting to be effective and purposeful?
- What are the desired outcomes from the meeting?
- What is a good time to hold the meeting? How much advance notice will people require in order to be able to attend?

- Where is the best place to hold it?
- What considerations must be made to enable participants to take part fully? For example, will a loop system be needed, or a palantypist or interpreter need to be present? Is there adequate provision for people to use laptops?
- Does the date clash with religious festivals or prayer times?
- What information needs to be circulated to participants before the meeting in order for them to come prepared?
- Who will take the notes/minutes of the meeting and circulate them afterwards? What is the agreed timescale for sending out the minutes?
- What amount of time is available for the meeting? When should it end?

## Preparing the agenda

It is important for you, as chair, to be very familiar with the shape and structure of the meeting, the order of the items and what actions or decisions are needed to flow from them.

If there are some difficult or contentious issues to be discussed, organise the agenda in such a way as to allow enough time for them. You may wish to allocate blocks of time to certain items. For example, you could suggest that after the first 30 minutes, you will move to the substantive item for discussion. This is a matter of judgement and forethought on your part as the chair, with prior consultation with other members as appropriate.

If the meeting is due to last for longer than say two hours, you need to have some agreement about comfort breaks in order to maximise people's concentration levels. Similarly, if refreshments are provided, you will need to agree when these are best taken to avoid unnecessary interruption.

In some organisations, there is a section on the agenda which is strictly confidential, which only certain designated members are allowed to share. This is an area where you as chair need to be very clear about the rules, and to make sure that they are strictly adhered to. It sometimes helps to announce a short break at this point to allow non-participating members to withdraw.

It is also worth annotating your own copy of the agenda with various points that you need to remember as the meeting progresses.

## The meeting itself

Many of the skills you will need to chair a meeting successfully are the same ones you need in your one-to-one interactions and interviews; it is just that they need to be adapted to a larger group setting. For example, you will want at the outset to ensure that you begin punctually, and to indicate how long the meeting is likely to last. You will need to introduce yourself and give any additional information about yourself that confirms your appropriateness as the chair of the meeting. You will then need to remind people of the purpose of the meeting, and what you are hoping to achieve. It is helpful also to remind people to turn off mobile phones/pagers, or to put them in silent mode.

Next, you need to invite people to introduce themselves and the capacity in which they are attending the meeting. This serves two functions: first, it enables everyone present to put faces to names; and second, it highlights the roles and responsibilities the agencies represented have to fulfil. In these days of increasing multi-agency cooperation, this is particularly important.

*Matters arising* are important. There may be action points from the previous meeting that need to be reported on, with the outcome noted in the minutes. It is your responsibility as chair to identify these, and to ask the appropriate person to give a brief report on progress.

When you reach the substantive items on the agenda for discussion, you need to have a clear view about what outcome you are seeking to achieve. This will affect how you chair the meeting. For example, if the item is a free-flowing exchange of ideas about various ways in which the organisation can improve its image and profile with the general public, you may want people to have brief discussions in pairs to get them going, and then report their ideas back to the whole group. You may then want to suggest that a subgroup brings a considered set of recommendations to the next meeting.

By contrast, if there is a serious matter to be decided at the meeting itself, you will need to consider how best it should be introduced. It may be right for you to speak briefly about it, highlighting the arguments for and against; or you may have invited someone else in advance to do this for you. Whatever tactic you adopt, it is important that you ensure that all points of view are clearly articulated in the discussion. Inevitably, some members may be more vociferous than others, so you will need from time to time to invite those who have not yet spoken to share their views in the meeting. You may do this in a general way, or speak directly to someone and ask them if they have anything they wish to add to the discussion. This needs to be done in a sensitive way, but you need to be seen as a chair who is even-handed and values the contribution which everyone can make to the debate.

Undoubtedly, one of the most difficult skills to learn is how to keep a discussion focused. It is your task as chair to keep the discussion on track without appearing rude or domineering. If you do not do this, there is bound to be a growing feeling that the real purpose of the meeting is not being achieved. One useful 'trick of the trade' is to thank people for their contributions so far, to remind them of what the main issues are that they need to decide on, and to draw their attention to aspects of the topic that have not yet been discussed. Towards the end, you can ask if anyone else wishes to contribute before you call for a vote. In extreme cases, you will need to be very assertive and to remind people of the ground rules whereby they agree to listen to each other without interruption, and to avoid being domineering. On occasion, you may need to address the person who is being domineering, thanking them for making their point so clearly, but asking them to sit back for a while to allow other members of the group to put their points forward.

You may also be surprised about how effective some appropriate hand gestures can be. If, for example, you look clearly at someone whom you wish to invite to speak and point to them, and at the same time hold your other hand up with the palm facing in the direction of the person whom you want to stay quiet, you are giving a message about your authority as chair.

**C**

Your role as chair also involves keeping an eye on the clock. When you feel that the issues have been sufficiently aired, announce that you intend to take the vote very soon. This helps people focus their thoughts on the key themes of the debate, and also provides a final opportunity for anyone who has not yet contributed to have their say.

## Voting

You need to record carefully those who vote *for*, those who vote *against* and those who *abstain*. You should then formally announce the decision of the meeting. You must be aware, however, of any constitutional regulations in this matter. Some organisations constitutionally require a 75 per cent majority in favour, for example, before any major change can be implemented. The group should be reminded of such regulations at the outset of the discussion and before the vote is taken. If it is a large group, you may wish to appoint two tellers to take responsibility for counting the votes.

Another point to bear in mind is eligibility to vote. There are some organisations where there is a strict membership entitlement to vote, and there needs to be a mechanism to ensure that non-voting people at the meeting clearly understand this rule. This is sometimes achieved by issuing voting papers, especially in cases where people are being elected to office.

The nightmare scenario for any chair, of course, is an evenly balanced vote. Sometimes the chair is allowed an additional casting vote, and it may be important that you exercise this. However, there is wisdom in thinking twice before you do this. Sometimes it is better simply to note that the meeting is so divided that you will need to return to the discussion next time. But there will be occasions when you will have to cast that deciding vote. If you do take that course of action, you should state your reasons for your decision. It is not easy or comfortable territory, but the chair has to fulfil this role effectively if business is to be conducted in due order.

## Involving service users, carers or patients in meetings

One further area demands particular skills from you as chair. Increasingly, there are meetings within health and social care settings where service users and carers and patients/relatives are involved in discussions and debates with professionals about their welfare, including the resources that are allocated to them. In such situations, as chair you will need to ensure, in advance of the meeting, that mentors or advocates will attend to support service users and carers who might feel intimidated by a powerful array of professionals.

Your role as chair is crucial in welcoming people and helping to put them at ease. You will need to remind them that specific time and space will be given to listening to their point of view, both directly and if necessary through their advocate. You will want everyone to feel that this is a genuine commitment, so that, whatever the outcome, they will feel that they have been properly listened to and their concerns fully heard.

Of course, there will be occasions when service users have no hesitation in voicing their concerns angrily and vociferously at the meeting. Your role will then be to encourage them directly, and with the support of their advocate if need be, to also listen to what others have to say. This is not easy; sometimes you may need to adjourn the meeting for a 5- or 10-minute 'comfort break' to allow tempers to calm down, and for you to speak to people informally. If, however, you can identify the fears and concerns that underlie people's contributions to the discussion, it will go a long way to helping the group come to its decision. If everyone respects your calm and authoritative role as chair, it will help them move towards a successful conclusion.

## Endings

It is important when you enter 'injury time' in a meeting – this is the period of about 15 minutes before its scheduled time for completion – that you draw people's attention to the time, and to the items still remaining for discussion. It is helpful sometimes to check to see if people can stay a further 30 minutes to complete the agenda. If they can, well and good, and you need to respect that revised timetable. If, however, people have to leave, then you need to agree what can be left until next time.

## Any other business?

There are various approaches to the mysterious item on many agendas: Any other business (AOB). As chair, you will need to exercise some judgement about any items that are raised. If they are fairly straightforward and can be dealt with in the time remaining, then there is no reason why you should not deal with them there and then. But if they require longer debate, or appear to be contentious or even mischievous, you should rule that they be placed on the agenda for the next meeting so that people have adequate notice.

## Date of the next meeting

It is not unusual for the trickiest discussion to focus around the date for the next meeting. If you are involved in a committee which has to meet regularly throughout the year, it is helpful to set the dates for the next six or so meetings well in advance.

Before you close the meeting formally, remember to thank people for their attendance and their contributions.

## Debriefing

If chairing meetings is still new to you, you may well find it helpful to have a debriefing discussion with a more experienced colleague to identify what went well, and to feed back ways in which you might have handled certain parts of the meeting differently. This will help you develop your confidence.

You will also find that you are beginning to watch other people's skills and techniques in chairing meetings where you are a participant. It is good to have some role models to help you develop your own particular skills, and it can be reassuring to see how even experienced chairs can, from time to time, struggle in this role.

Finally, you need to arrange to meet with the person taking the minutes to ensure that they are accurate and ready in time to send out to members before the next meeting.

### Minute taking

Many organisations have secretarial support for taking minutes, but from time to time you may be called upon to fulfil this role. It goes without saying that the accuracy of minutes and notes of meetings is of vital importance. People who lead busy lives and attend many meetings may well not remember the details of the discussions and the decisions taken at each one, so the record of the meeting is crucial. For committees and groups that meet on a regular basis, these ongoing records are the only means whereby the story of what is decided is accurately told. Future members of the committee may need to look back on the minutes from several years back to check certain facts and decisions. So the minutes need to be accurate, agreed by the committee meeting members and stored safely but accessibly, in hard copy as well as electronically, for all who have good reason to consult them.

You also need to decide on the style of minutes appropriate to your meeting. Sometimes all that is needed is a set of action points or decisions, but on other occasions a more detailed account of the issues that were discussed is necessary. There may also be confidential items that should not appear in the general minutes but need recording elsewhere.

---

### Group exercise

With the help of your tutor or supervisor, devise a scenario for a multi-disciplinary case conference, either based on your own experience or it could be fictitious. Decide how many professional roles need to be present and discuss the arguments and positions each one will take in the meeting. Agree who is to be the chair, and run the scenario. Allow time for pauses during the role play to help guide and support the chair, with opportunity for others to practise their chairing skills. After the meeting has been concluded, discuss as a group the challenges and skills needed to chair such meetings effectively.

---

## FINAL THOUGHTS

This discussion has highlighted the importance of detailed planning, preparation and good communication skills in the context of chairing meetings and recording the decisions and outcomes. If as chair you can develop the necessary communication skills to help people work together in meetings to debate difficult issues and come to clear decisions, you will have made a significant contribution to the organisations involved.

## REFERENCES AND FURTHER READING

Honey, P. (2004) *How to Chair Meetings Effectively*. Maidenhead: Peter Honey.
Hugman, B. (2009) *Healthcare Communication*. London: Pharmaceutical Press.
Kelsey, D. and Plumb, P. (2004) *Great Meetings! Great Results. A Practical Guide for Facilitating Successful Productive Meetings*. Portland, ME: Great Meetings Inc.

**RELATED CONCEPTS** feedback (giving and receiving); interpreters; non-verbal-communication

**ENGAGING WITH THE PCF** context and organisations; professional leadership; professionalism

**ENGAGING WITH THE NMC CODE** promote professionalism and trust

### Service user snippet

Jay (21), social work student:

'When my supervisor told me I had to chair an important team meeting as part of my training my legs turned to jelly. Fortunately, I studied the entry in Moss' *Communication Skills* and that helped me prepare properly. It was still a scary experience but I coped!' (Personal email)

# CHALLENGING

The ability to challenge inappropriate or offensive language or behaviour in others is one of the most difficult communication skills to put into practice. Often you feel caught between the 'rock' of doing or saying nothing and thereby appearing to collude with the other person, and the 'hard place' of over-reacting and making matters worse by provoking or alienating the other person and losing the thread of the discussion which you were trying to hold with them.

Part of the reason for this, perhaps, lies in the word itself. 'Challenging' seems to be a very aggressive activity, highly 'macho' and confrontational: very much 'in your face', as we might say. Certainly, in some of the early examples of anti-racist awareness training, an openly confrontational approach was often deemed necessary by some of the trainers in order to bring white people up with a jolt, and make them realise just how serious and ingrained racism is within a white-dominated society. Many people-workers may feel very uncomfortable about being expected to adopt such a style or approach, however worthy the intention might be; it seems to smack too much of adopting the moral high ground in our relationship with others.

Just because it is difficult, however, does not mean that you should give up the attempt. Challenging is an important activity for you because it goes to the very heart of the value base of the work you undertake with others. The values of dignity, respect, social justice and celebrating diversity are central to your work, but they do not come automatically or easily. Indeed, they often need to be championed against considerable opposition, as many events in the early part of the twenty-first century so eloquently testify. Challenging opposing sets of values is important precisely because of this struggle: if prejudice and discriminatory practice are not challenged, it is one further tiny victory for intolerance and bigotry. But unavoidably this also makes demands upon your personal and professional assertiveness skills which may take you some time to develop, especially in the early stages of your career. Supervision and feedback therefore are valuable to help you grow in confidence.

## Activity

Spend a few moments jotting down some examples of statements or behaviour which you feel would be important for you to challenge. Keep these to hand while this discussion unfolds.

It is likely that your examples will feature some of the major social attitudes that have become contemporary 'isms': racism, sexism, classism, disablism and heterosexism, as well as homophobia, Islamophobia, and prejudices against LGBTI+ individuals and groups. Characteristics and differences that are seen by some to enrich our society are regarded by others with fear, suspicion and hostility. That each and every individual is capable of acting badly towards others is a sad feature of our human existence: it is when groups of people are labelled as 'deviant' or 'unacceptable' simply by their belonging to that group that we enter dangerous territory, where the importance of challenging becomes imperative.

## STYLES OF CHALLENGING

We must state at the outset that for all its aggressive potential, challenging as an activity can have quite a different 'feel' to it. It can be subtle or gentle; it can draw on humour or be accomplished non-verbally. Challenging, in other words, can often be achieved elegantly without the confrontation that many people so dislike.

Not all challenging is on a 'one-to-one' basis. Citizens Advice, for example, have an important social policy arm whereby issues that arise from individual enquirers which are seen to affect larger numbers of people are brought together into a campaigning activity. Pressure is brought to bear on local or national government to raise their awareness, and to seek some amelioration. Other examples of pressure groups such as the Child Poverty Action Group and various homeless charities provide similar examples of ways in which challenging can be achieved through campaigning to improve the quality of people's lives.

On an individual level, several options are open to you when faced with language and behaviour that is offensive. The most straightforward approach is calmly but firmly to ask the person to stop behaving or speaking in this way because you find it unacceptable. You need to find the best form of words to use, of course, but if you can own the discomfort and upset that this causes it will enable you to challenge it. It is even more helpful if your organisation has a policy about such matters. You can then draw people's attention to this and ask them not to talk or behave like that when on your premises.

Challenging, however, is rarely straightforward. Sometimes, in the middle of a difficult interview, someone may use language that you find offensive. You may well feel, however, that to interrupt the flow of the interview by making an immediate challenge would be too disruptive to the main purpose of the interview. In such circumstances, you may well simply make a mental note of this, and when the interview is winding down, gently refer to the incident and ask the person not to talk like that with you again.

It is useful to have some responses already prepared, or at least thought through, so that you do not always have to struggle to find the best form of words to use. Some examples of this include:

- 'I don't think we can say that these days, do you?'
- 'That really makes me feel uncomfortable when you say/do that.'
- 'I can't agree with what you have just said.'
- 'I don't think it is right to label everybody like that.'

- 'When people come to this office, we do ask everyone, including the staff, to be careful about the language we all use so that we don't cause offence.'

The key issue is that you are not necessarily inviting a debate about the subject, although from time to time that may be helpful and appropriate and will help you to discuss the value base you are working from. The important thing is that you are making clear how you feel about their discriminatory or offensive language and behaviour; you are owning and acknowledging the negative impact it has on you; you are naming it, and are reinforcing the boundaries within which you find it acceptable to work with this person.

Many agencies have statements about language and behaviour clearly on view for everyone to see. For people who cannot read, other ways of putting this message across need to be found – pictorial representations are useful alternatives here. In the last resort, you would be entitled to draw your meeting to a close and to refuse to work any further with the person if their offensive behaviour or language persisted. In such situations, it is a good idea to warn them that you feel unable to continue, but to ask them to wait so that you can bring in your manager to reinforce the point and to support you. All being well, the person will then modify their behaviour, but if they do need to be excluded from the agency, you will then have had appropriate support for this course of action.

If you do need to take this drastic action, it is helpful to follow it up with a letter explaining the reason for your decision, and offering them a further appointment on the strict understanding that next time they should observe the ground rules you have established. This gives them a chance to reflect and to make a fresh start.

Sometimes, of course, this sort of behaviour is the result of someone being heavily under the influence of alcohol or affected by drugs misuse. It is wise to call an early halt to any such interview, and ask them to return for a further appointment when they are in full control of themselves. You should not be expected to put yourself in a risky, vulnerable situation by continuing an interview with someone whose self-control is in question. Nor is it fair to expect a person who is not in full control of themselves to engage in discussion or work on key issues that affect their lives. In some settings, however, such as hospitals, it may be necessary to summon help from security colleagues if a person's behaviour constitutes a risk to others. As a last resort, in hostels or residential settings, for example, the police may have to be called in order to respect and maintain the safety of others. In such cases, you need clearly and calmly to ask the person concerned to moderate their language or behaviour, and to advise them that if they refuse to comply or to leave the premises, the police will be called.

## Group exercise

With the help of your tutor or supervisor, identify a number of scenarios where you feel you would need to challenge someone, and make a list of possible responses. Then, within your group, work in pairs to practise your responses. By doing this in a safe group environment, with support from your tutor or supervisor, you will develop confidence in this important area.

## Challenging and other professionals

Much of what we have said above is relevant across the board, especially if you encounter oppressive, abusive language or behaviour, but there may be particularly difficult moments when you find yourself wondering how to challenge a fellow professional face to face or in a meeting where there are divergent views being expressed. This can be even more difficult if the person you need to challenge is in a more senior position than you, or represents another profession. In a nursing context, being a junior member of staff trying to challenge a ward sister or even a consultant may always feel a step too far unless their value base is such that they actively welcome shared decision making and debate.

Perhaps the hardest part is 'keeping your cool', trying not to be flustered by the daunting prospect of launching the challenge. Sometimes it helps to have a form of words ready to use to help open up the dialogue between you. For example, try this for size:

'I appreciate where you are coming from J, but can we look at it another way for a moment please?'

'To be honest J, I hadn't considered that point of view before. I was approaching it from another angle.'

'To be honest J, I'm wondering how the service user/patient would feel about your approach to this? Might there be some merit in looking at it from another perspective?'

Of course, there is no guarantee that any one verbal formula will do the trick: the power dynamics between you may always get in the way. But you will have made your point as a fellow professional that your opinion and professional judgement deserve to be taken into account, especially in an interprofessional context. Sometimes the ultimate responsibility for a decision may not rest with you, but so long as you feel you have contributed to the consideration of the issues you will have done what you can. At such moments you may be left feeling disappointed, frustrated or let down, so it is important that you record the episode clearly in relevant documentation and raise it in supervision, especially if you feel your professionally considered opinion has been ignored.

There may be times also when you are on the receiving end of challenging comments from other professionals, which can have a very demoralising impact upon you. Again, the golden rule is to 'keep your cool'; listen respectfully, and find ways of putting your point of view across. Maybe they have a point that you hadn't fully considered; maybe you feel they are just wanting to 'put you down'. Whatever the circumstances, it is important that you behave professionally and with dignity and keep to the forefront of your mind what is in the service user/patient's best interest. If afterwards you feel you have been disrespectfully treated, harassed or bullied, you should raise this in supervision, and actively consider whether whistleblowing or making a complaint is justified. There will be occasions where it is appropriate for you to arrange to meet with the other professional afterwards, with a colleague present, to discuss the issue and raise your concerns. This may take courage, and we all need to think carefully about which battles must be fought; but you may be pleasantly surprised by the outcome. You are a professional – not a door mat!

## FINAL THOUGHTS

'All it takes for evil to flourish is for good people to do nothing.' If we apply this principle to our present discussion, we will see that even the smallest, very low-key challenge may make an important impact.

## REFERENCES AND FURTHER READING

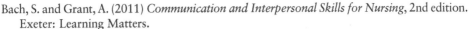

Bach, S. and Grant, A. (2011) *Communication and Interpersonal Skills for Nursing*, 2nd edition. Exeter: Learning Matters.
Egan, G. (2017) *The Skilled Helper: A Client Centred Approach*, 2nd EMEA edition. Chicago, IL: Cengage Learning.
Thompson, N. (2011) *Effective Communication*, 2nd edition. Basingstoke: Palgrave Macmillan.
Trevithick, P. (2012) *Social Work Skills: A Practice Handbook*, 3rd edition. Maidenhead: Open University Press.

**RELATED CONCEPTS** anti-discriminatory practice; assertiveness; barrier gestures; conflict management; empathy; endings

**ENGAGING WITH THE PCF** contexts and organisations; critical reflection and analysis; diversity; skills and interventions; professionalism

**ENGAGING WITH THE NMC CODE** prioritise people; promote professionalism and trust

### Service user snippet

Mandeep (19), nursing student:

'When I heard this consultant slagging off a Muslim patient on our ward, I nearly died with embarrassment. It took me all my courage to say "Excuse me, but I didn't think you should say things like that". It was so difficult but I was so angry – he should not have said what he said. But afterwards, to give him his due, he thanked me and apologised. But will he do it again? I'm not sure. But what more can I do?'

# COMPLAINTS

Our attitude towards complaints tells us a lot about our values and those of our workplace. Some organisations positively welcome complaints because they want to constantly be improving the quality of the service they offer. Others seem to regard complaints almost as a personal insult and will go to any lengths to ignore them or to make the person bringing the complaint feel guilty or that they are a timewaster.

## Activity

Think for a moment of when you have needed to make a complaint, perhaps in a restaurant, shop or hospital. How were you treated? How did this experience make you feel?

Your reactions to this Activity will be revealing. If you were treated respectfully, listened to carefully and promised some action, you will most likely have felt relieved and glad that you had taken the trouble. If, on the other hand, you were ignored, put down and dealt with dismissively, you will most likely have felt angry, hurt and made to suspect that the organisation is trying to cover up its mistakes. In a compensation-active society, the temptation for people to cover their backs is huge. In the care industry we have seen many examples of this: Stafford Hospital was but one of a series of shameful cases of neglect that came to light, not least because people had the courage to complain and to take on large organisations in the search for truth (Francis, 2013). For a further discussion of this aspect of complaints, please see *Whistleblowing*.

We will focus now on best practice guidelines when dealing with people who wish to make a complaint.

The first thing to emphasise is that you need to be aware of the complaints procedures adopted by your organisation, and who is the key person to whom complaints should be addressed. You may have a formal complaints form to give to people, although sometimes people prefer to have the matter dealt with informally. The clearer you can be about your organisation's policy and procedures, the easier it will be for you to deal with.

There are some very straightforward responses you can use which make all the difference and often can help to defuse a tense situation. These can be summed up in four responses: 'thank you', 'glad', 'sorry', 'sure'.

*Thank you*: It may come as a real surprise to the person making the complaint to be thanked for taking the time and trouble to raise their concerns. They may have been expecting defensiveness, hostility even, but a calm '*thank you for bringing this to our attention – thank you for taking the trouble to come and tell us about this*' immediately conveys the message that you are taking the matter seriously and treating them with courtesy and respect.

*Glad*: This strengthens and underlines the sincerity of your approach. '*I am glad you have brought this to our attention*' will almost be music to the ears of the person who has plucked up the courage to make the complaint. Even with people who are initially aggressive and bombastic in their approach, demanding to have something done, this calm, professional, non-defensive approach is effective.

*Sorry*: Used carefully, the expression '*I am sorry*' takes the process one step further. '*I am sorry you have had this experience – I am sorry this has happened to you*' reinforces your commitment to take this matter seriously. We say 'use this carefully' because it is not appropriate to start taking sides or agreeing that the complaint is justified. It may not be; it may be a vendetta or a malicious attempt to attack someone's reputation. But it is appropriate to express some empathy.

*Sure*: The final step is to give assurance to the person making the complaint that it will be dealt with by the appropriate person in the organisation in a thorough, professional manner. '*I am sure that the manager will deal with this – I am sure that you will receive a response and that it will be properly investigated.*' This is the point at which you can clarify how best to proceed. Would the person like to wait to see if you can find a manager to talk with them? Would they like to make an appointment for another occasion? Would they like to take the complaints form and bring it back duly completed? Would they like help in filling in the form? Each case will be different and you will need to exercise sensitivity and discretion. But in the end you hope that when the discussion ends they will feel you have dealt with them respectfully, and that the complaint will be taken seriously. You need also to ensure that they are very clear about what happens next in the process, how they will be communicated with about the outcome, and whether they will need to be prepared to come back to give more details as part of the investigative process.

## Group exercise

With the help of your tutor or supervisor, identify some recent examples of complaints made to your organisation or professional body. How do you think they were handled? What lessons can you learn from these examples to inform your own professional practice?

## FINAL THOUGHTS

How you respond to complaints provides a powerful litmus test for the culture of your organisation. If you can gratefully welcome a genuine complaint and recognise its potential to improve the service you offer, you will enhance your commitment to best practice.

## REFERENCES AND FURTHER READING

Francis, R. (2013) *Report of the Mid Staffordshire NHS Foundation Trust Public Inquiry.* Norwich: TSO.
Trevithick, P. (2012) *Social Work Skills and Knowledge: A Practice Handbook*, 3rd edition. Maidenhead: Open University Press.

**RELATED CONCEPTS** assertiveness; dealing with upset service users; whistleblowing

**ENGAGING WITH THE PCF** contexts and organisations; skills and interventions; professional leadership; professionalism

**ENGAGING WITH THE NMC CODE** promote professionalism and trust

### Service user snippet

Jaswinder (20), nursing student:

'I couldn't believe the awful neglect in mum's nursing home. I was shocked, to tell you the truth, and when I tried to talk to the staff they just said how busy they were and in any case it was none of my business. Fortunately, I knew about complaints procedures and the ombudsman from my training course so I told them that was what I would do. I think that shook them a bit. But you've got to do it haven't you – they can't get away with neglecting people in their care, can they?'

# CONFIDENTIALITY

In almost all aspects of professional people-work, the principle of confidentiality is highlighted as part of the value base and the various codes of practice. If people feel that their privacy will be violated by the person they speak to, or their personal details made public in some way, they will not have confidence in the service they are being offered. Nor will the relationship that is being offered to them be regarded as professional. So it is extremely important that people are reassured at the outset about this central tenet of professional people-work: they need to know where they are before they can begin to trust the person they are working with.

This general principle, however, is not as straightforward as some would think.

---

## Activity

Think about the organisation you work for, or an agency you are familiar with. What information is given to your service users/clients/patients about confidentiality? What are the particular aspects of confidentiality that are central to your work? Are there any boundaries to confidentiality? If so, what are they, and how are these boundaries explained to people?

---

This exercise will have revealed that confidentiality is rarely, if ever, absolute. Agencies recognise that there are sometimes overriding societal responsibilities laid upon them which would mean that an individual's right to confidentiality must be compromised. For example, if information is divulged which indicates that a vulnerable person – a child or an adult – is being put at risk, or is being abused or harmed in any way, then there is a duty laid upon the worker to report that information. This would be done first of all within the agency to an appropriate senior manager, and then if necessary to another agency, such as the police or social workers, charged with a role of protecting vulnerable people.

This has been a topic which has posed a particular challenge for leaders in faith-based organisations, where traditionally the 'priest's confessional' (or its equivalent) has been regarded as absolute. In recent years, however, there has been an increasing awareness of the overriding duty to protect vulnerable children in particular. Faith groups have been taking urgent steps, therefore, to ensure that they respect this moral and legal imperative; to have in place policies and procedures to safeguard vulnerable children and adults, and, where necessary, to report all cases of abuse to the police. Stories that emerge of historic sex abuse, especially towards children and vulnerable young people, illustrate the corrosive power of cover-ups that protected the abuser and left the abused unheard, unsupported and unbelieved.

---

### Group exercise

With the help of your tutor or supervisor, choose a recent example of historic sex abuse, in a secular or religious context, that has been reported in the press. What were the key issues being highlighted? As a group draw up some 'bullet points' for best practice, outlining your recommendations to help prevent such abuse happening again, with particular focus on implications for confidentiality.

---

One fundamental point to stress is that confidentiality is both an organisational and an individual commitment. From the individual worker's perspective, there is a commitment that information will not be divulged to other people outside the organisation except in very exceptional circumstances. Trevithick (2012: 292) reminds us, however, that 'in keeping with the requirements of the Data Protection Act 1998, it is important for service users to know what information is being passed between one agency and another ... and who has access to their records.' But this commitment does not mean that the information will not be shared within the organisation: it is of crucial importance that managers are aware of what is happening, so that they can advise the worker on the best action to take, especially if sensitive information is being handled.

Confidentiality has important implications when poor or harmful practice occurs. Loyalty to colleagues must not override your obligations to best practice and the duty you have to raise these concerns in an appropriate manner, if necessary through whistleblowing. One of the results of the Francis Report into the Mid Staffordshire NHS Trust (Francis, 2013) has been the introduction of the duty of candour, which lays a legal duty on healthcare organisations in England to be open and honest with patients when harm has been caused. This principle deserves to be respected in all people-work so that the people who come to you for help can be confident that mistakes will not be covered up but will be dealt with openly, honestly and effectively.

## GENERAL DATA PROTECTION REGULATION

The introduction of the General Data Protection Regulation (GDPR) in May 2018 (ICO, 2018) has had far-reaching effects on each and every organisation that holds other people's data and information. Its aim is clear: any organisation needs to have specific permission to hold data on anyone who is in any way connected with them. Without this specific written permission organisations should delete any previous personal information they hold on people and should not communicate with them in future.

Needless to say, this new regulation has also had far-reaching consequences, leading also to come confusion about what compliance really means. Compliance is a responsibility for individual workers as well as their employers. What you keep in your diary or on your mobile phone or laptop comes under the purview of the legislation. In other words, GDPR is an individual professional as well as an organisational imperative.

All we can do here, of course, is to signpost you to the implications of GDPR for your own organisation. You have a responsibility to understand how this legislation impacts upon your professional practice; what procedures you need to follow, and how data is safely protected and stored. You also need to be familiar with your organisation's procedures for informing people for whom you have a responsibility of care how the requirements of GDPR are being implemented.

## RAISING THE ISSUE

This book focuses on communication skills, and does not attempt a full-scale discussion of complex issues which can be found elsewhere in the literature. The key challenge for you as a people-worker, therefore, is how you can most effectively raise the issue of confidentiality with the people with whom you are working.

As so often in people-work, there is no single form of words that you must always use. Each of you must find a way of tackling these issues and a form of words that you feel comfortable with using. The following suggestion is designed only to get you thinking and to find the best way you can explain these important issues:

'It's good to see you today, J. Before we go any further, I need to explain a few things to you about confidentiality. I hope you realise that we will deal with you with the utmost respect and that what you say to us will not go outside this office unless in very exceptional circumstances. One of the ways in which we try to give you the best possible service is to ensure that I as a (student/ worker/nurse) can seek guidance and advice from my manager/supervisor, and this is what I will be doing with the work we will be doing together.'

'But there will be occasions with some people, J, when they tell us things which we then have to do something about. The sort of thing I mean is when we hear about children or vulnerable adults being abused or put at risk. If we hear about that sort of thing, we are legally bound to inform social workers or the police, so that they can investigate, and I am sure you appreciate the importance of that. Other than that, J, we would always seek your consent before we spoke to anyone else about you. And even if we felt we had to contact someone else, we would always tell you what we were going to have to do. I'm sorry if this sounds a bit long-winded, J, but I hope you understand how important it is. Would you like to tell me how you now understand these issues?'

'May I ask you, J, if you have heard of the recent change in the law about data protection? It is called the General Data Protection Regulation and is intended to keep everyone's personal information safe and secure. What it means for us is that we need your permission to keep in touch with you. Are you happy for us to do this?'

## On a personal note

The discussion so far has focused on your professional obligations towards those with whom you work to ensure that information is handled appropriately and respectfully, and that you understand the boundaries to confidentiality. There is, however, a further dimension which deserves attention, and this is about the obligation you have towards yourself as a professional worker. You will be bound by professional codes of conduct, which have implications for your private life as well as how you perform at work. If you have a criminal record, for example, you are likely to be deemed unsuitable for many aspects of people-work. Much as you might wish to keep some personal details secret and confidential, you are under an obligation to inform your manager about any aspect of your private life which can reasonably be assumed to impact upon your professional performance and/or the reputation of your agency.

In some ways, this also includes how you engage with the various social networking sites that have become so central to people's interactive communications. Once you have put some information or some personal photographs onto your social networking site, they are likely to be there for some time, even though recent developments now allow you to remove certain material. Furthermore, not all sites are completely secure, which means that an unscrupulous person could make an entry on your behalf that you would totally disown, or send on to others material that you would not wish to have widely disseminated. This is not to suggest that as a professional people-worker you should not use social networking sites, but it is a gentle note of caution to urge you to take care when using them, and to always ask whether the material you are putting onto the site would in any way compromise your professional integrity. This is why some professionals use fictitious names on social media sites in order to protect themselves. But photographs rarely lie, so the utmost caution must always be applied when uploading 'selfies'.

### Group exercise

With the help of your tutor or supervisor, as a group consider each of the following scenarios. Identify the issues and potential dilemmas for confidentiality.

1   You notice a colleague delivering poor practice: whom, if anyone, should you tell?
2   The local press ring you for a comment on one of your clients who has been in trouble.

3 A local GP rings you to discuss one of your service users.
4 You need information from a local school about a young person whom you suspect of 'drug pushing'.
5 A service user tells you about their nextdoor neighbour who is 'always making their toddler cry'.
6 You work at your local hospital and see signs of neglect on the wards.
7 You serve on a local committee which has decided, against your advice, to close down a local residential care home for people with dementia. You are invited to serve on the local 'save our care home' campaign.

## FINAL THOUGHTS

Confidentiality is one of the core values of all people-work; it will repay some careful attention so that you are completely familiar with your agency's policies, procedures and expectations, and that you are comfortable with how you explain these to others.

## REFERENCES AND FURTHER READING

Brammer, A. (2020) *Social Work Law*, 5th edition. Harlow: Pearson.
Clarke, C. (2000) *Social Work Ethics: Politics, Principles and Practice*. Basingstoke: Macmillan.
Francis, R. (2013) *Report of the Mid Staffordshire NHS Foundation Trust Public Inquiry*. Norwich: TSO.
Hugman, R. (2005) *New Approaches in Ethics for the Caring Professions*. Basingstoke: Palgrave Macmillan.
Information Commissioner's Office (ICO) (2018) *Guide to the General Data Protection Regulation (GDPR)*. Wilmslow: ICO.
Trevithick, P. (2012) *Social Work Skills: A Practice Handbook*, 3rd edition. Maidenhead: Open University Press.

**RELATED CONCEPTS** communication and social media; establishing a professional relationship; non-verbal communication; supervision; whistleblowing

**ENGAGING WITH THE PCF** contexts and organisations; interprofessional collaboration; professionalism; values and ethics

**ENGAGING WITH THE NMC CODE** prioritise people; promote professionalism and trust

### Service user snippet

John (22), social work student:

'He seemed so plausible when he rang me up asking about his elderly relative who was on my caseload. So I told him all about her ... it was only afterwards that the panic set in. I hadn't checked who I was talking to or whether he was bona fide. I'll never make that mistake again.'

# CONFLICT MANAGEMENT

Conflict is at the very heart of people-work, especially for professionals such as social workers, police and probation officers, who are often required to balance individual rights and freedoms against risks and harm to others. The very act of undertaking a risk assessment on an individual or family carries with it the likelihood of decisions being taken with which some of the people involved may violently disagree. To remove a child 'at risk' from a family to a place of safety, or to insist that someone in mental distress goes into hospital for treatment, is to be involved in conflict. Within a multi-disciplinary hospital team, there could also be conflicting approaches to how to work most effectively with, or treat, a particular individual or family. Most people-workers and healthcare workers can also give examples of times when they have had to deal with angry, distressed or disappointed people whose response has often provoked high levels of conflict. To develop appropriate communication skills for dealing with conflict is, therefore, essential.

It is worth pausing for a moment to take stock of just how pervasive this theme of conflict is within people-work.

## Activity

Jot down as many examples as you can think of where conflict has occurred in your workplace, or in a setting where you have been involved as a student or trainee. Note what the issues were, who was involved and how it made the various people feel. Also try to identify the power issues involved.

Your list will probably be quite a long one, and as this discussion unfolds it will be useful to refer back to it from time to time.

One of the first things to note is that conflict need not necessarily be a bad thing. We have all come across organisations and teams of people who have become comfortable, even complacent, in how they are performing and fulfilling their tasks and roles. If we are honest, most of us prefer 'a quiet life' where we can get on with things in a familiar way, and to have fixed and familiar routines can be of tremendous help when workloads escalate. But best practice, informed by relevant research, means that we need to be challenged and stretched, and this is not always a comfortable experience. A new manager may see things in a different light, and new policies and procedures may be introduced specifically to improve the agency's service delivery. In such situations, conflict may be seen as a positive experience, as new ways of working come into conflict with older methods within an overall commitment to improve the quality of the services being provided.

Nevertheless, conflict is a complex issue. If you refer to your list from the above Activity, you may well have included examples of conflict in the following areas:

- You may find yourself 'at odds' with your manager/organisation about the best way of dealing with certain situations.
- You may face an internal conflict within yourself over a moral or ethical issue and how you are expected to behave at work – dealing with abortion or drug misuse, for example.
- You may vehemently disagree with national or local government policy in an area of work with which you are involved – implementing cuts in services, for example, or how most effectively to supervise serious offenders in the community.
- You may 'fall out' with a colleague at work due to a personality clash or difference of opinion.
- Your team may be split in its opinions about how best to proceed on a certain issue.
- You may be called upon to take, or to support, industrial action against your employer.
- Your service user may have strongly differing opinions about what is the best thing for you both to do when tackling certain problems.

These are a few snapshots of the world of conflict that is at the heart of people-work. In all of them, you will no doubt have to take decisions that are difficult, and you certainly will not be able to please all of the people all of the time. But the fact remains that it is not just the decisions that are important – it is also crucial to practise the communication skills that will be needed to implement them.

As always, core communication skills are essential in such situations. When conflict involves your work with service users or carers, then the following 'golden rules' always apply:

- Be open and honest and clear in what you are doing, and explain clearly why you are doing it.
- Remind people that they have the right not just of reply but of challenging you through appropriate channels.
- See people face to face, and allow them the opportunity to voice their concerns, however vociferously. Ensure that these views are recorded, with a copy given to them for their information.

It is also helpful to have a framework within which to work when handling conflict. This will give you an added confidence in dealing with stressful situations. Thompson (2012) has suggested what he calls the *RED approach* to managing conflict. In this framework, *R* stands for *recognising* the conflict. This seems an obvious point to make, but unless the conflict is recognised and named as such, there is a risk that it will not be tackled. We are all familiar with a general sense of unease, or a feeling that all is not quite as it should be, and often we ignore it and hope that it will go away. The act of acknowledging that this is due to a conflict is an important first step towards dealing with it. In his discussion of this point, Thompson (2012: 184ff) also reminds us of the tendency we have to individualise difficulties and to regard the 'other people' as being difficult or uncooperative, whereas the truth may lie elsewhere in a much broader context.

*E* requires us to *evaluate* the conflict. Few of us wish to be constantly on the lookout for trouble, and one of the skills of our job is to know when to deal with an issue 'head-on' and when to leave it well alone. The key point here, however, is the importance of making that decision, and coming to a view about how serious or otherwise the conflict really is. Without doubt, if it is serious and is disregarded, then the chances of it festering and gradually worsening are high. The evaluation of conflict requires us to try to get behind the behaviours and language of the people concerned, and to gain as clear a picture as possible about what the conflict is really about. This will enable us to take the third and final step of *dealing* with it (*D*).

Thompson warns us against the twin dangers of (1) an ostrich-like 'head in the sand' ignoring of the problem altogether, and, by contrast, (2) an over-reaction which can escalate and exacerbate the difficulties. It is in the *appropriate* dealing with the conflict that real communication skills lie. In some situations, mediation skills may be useful to help people in dispute work towards a resolution. As a general rule, however, it is important to feel comfortable about taking the risk of asking people what the matter is, or saying that you sense something is wrong, or wondering if there is anything you can do to help ease the situation. These gentle 'opening' questions or statements may be sufficient to open the lines of communication, and to begin to tease out what the difficulties really are.

Once they become clear, of course, then a further evaluation will be needed to decide what action, if any, is necessary to resolve the problems that have been identified.

## Group exercise

With the help of your tutor or supervisor, revisit as a group your list of conflict situations from the above Activity. Choose one or two to work through in a group discussion, and explore how the RED approach could help you handle these situations differently.

## FINAL THOUGHTS

No one pretends that managing conflict is easy or stress-free – exactly the opposite is often the case, although it must also be said that some people seem to thrive on conflict and get a real 'buzz' from it. But if conflict is ignored, it is unlikely to go away, and if it festers it is likely to be even harder to handle when the bubble eventually bursts. What you are encouraged to do as a result of reading this entry, therefore, is not to assume that you will need a whole new range of specialised communication skills to deal with conflict. Instead, you are encouraged to be true to yourself, to be honest and open with yourself and others, and to use a framework such as the RED approach to enable you to apply your basic skills to the resolution of conflict.

But do remember: some conflicts can only be handled higher up the chain of command, and sometimes the only responsible thing to do is to report your concerns to your manager, supervisor, tutor or practice educator, and ask for them to deal with the issues at that level. You do not have to carry the full responsibility for conflict if it has wider implications for your team or organisation.

## REFERENCES AND FURTHER READING

Charlton, R. and Dewdney, M. (2014) *The Mediator's Handbook: Skills and Strategies for Practitioners*, 3rd edition. London: Sweet & Maxwell.

Egan, G. (2014) *The Skilled Helper*, 10th international edition. Chicago, IL: Cengage Learning.

Stewart, S. (1998) *Conflict Resolution: A Foundation Guide*. Winchester: Waterside Press.

Thompson, N. (2012) *The People Solutions Sourcebook*, 2nd edition. Basingstoke: Palgrave Macmillan.

**RELATED CONCEPTS** dealing with upset service users; mediation skills; non-verbal communication; reflective practice; supervision; whistleblowing

**ENGAGING WITH THE PCF** skills and interventions; professional leadership

**ENGAGING WITH THE NMC CODE** promote professionalism and trust

### Service user snippet

Gerry (38), social worker:

'I really hate conflict in a team – it "does my head in". I'm all for a quiet life, me. But in my last team I had to leave, it was so bad. Things were never said to your face, and important issues were never discussed openly. Two or three in the team did their own thing and no one challenged them. Even the manager colluded with them, so what chance did the rest of us have? In the end I couldn't hack it, and left.'

# COUNSELLING

There is a clear overlap between counselling, counselling skills and the great variety of activities within people-work, but it is of critical importance that you are clear about the distinctions between them. It is not appropriate to regard counselling as a woolly 'catch-all' activity that is part of every people-worker's toolkit; but it *is* wholly appropriate to expect all people-workers and nurses to use at least some counselling skills in their day-to-day work.

## Activity

Spend some time trying to define what you understand 'counselling' to mean. Then see how many different definitions you can find for this complex activity. You might want to undertake a Google search to help you do this. Can you identify common themes? How do these definitions help in clarifying or describing what you do with your service users?

One of the problems you may discover in this search is that counselling is often used in a generalised rather than a specific way, sometimes even as a synonym for advice. Students who fail their exams, for example, are often advised to go for academic counselling, by which it is meant that they need to seek academic guidance and advice on what they did wrong and how they could improve their performance. In-depth exploration of their deepest feelings and aspirations would not be on the agenda for such an encounter.

Feltham and Dryden have produced a definition which has proved popular in the literature. They describe counselling as being:

> A principled relationship characterised by the application of one or more psychological theories and a recognised set of communication skills, modified by experience, intuition and other interpersonal factors, to clients' intimate concerns, problems or aspirations. Its predominant ethos is one of facilitation rather than of advice-giving or coercion. It may be of very brief or long duration, take place in an organisational or private practice setting, and may or may not overlap with practical, medical and other matters of personal welfare. (1993: 6)

'Counselling', therefore, is a generic term, and there is a wide variety of approaches and styles that are now in common practice. These include the psychodynamic approach, which emphasises the importance of unconscious influences on how people behave; the humanist-existential approach, which encourages people to recognise and develop their potential and to exercise creative choices in how they live and behave; and the cognitive-behavioural approach which seeks to help people change their observable behaviours and ways of thinking that underpin the difficulties they are facing in their lives (Nelson-Jones, 2015: 5). Each of these main approaches or schools can also be subdivided into different styles of therapy, each of which has its own distinctive style or approach. To all of this we might also wish to add a faith community perspective, through which people seek to change their lifestyle and behaviours more accurately to reflect the teachings of their chosen faith in obedience to a Supreme Being/God/Allah.

This complexity of counselling approaches is not intended to bewilder you. It is helpful for you to be aware, however, of the range of help and in-depth therapies that are available to people, and to recognise the comprehensive training and expertise that practitioners in these disciplines need to acquire in order to practise effectively. Their common theme and purpose is to work with their clients to help them resolve sometimes deep-seated difficulties, clarify their hopes, fears and aspirations, and move into the future in a more positive and dynamic way as a result of this intervention.

## BOUNDARIES

It is also important that you know what your own professional limitations are, and when it is appropriate for you to refer someone to more specialist care. You need to be clear in your own mind, in whatever branch of people-work you are involved, about the boundaries of your knowledge and skills. This will be the point at which you will need to begin to assess seriously whether the person you are working with needs to be referred to another agency, where perhaps expert counselling help or therapy can be made available.

For example, you may be working in a criminal justice setting where you have the responsibility to work with offenders to address and modify their offending behaviour. This will involve using a range of skills and suggesting various strategies to help people control their anger or their abusive behaviour. If, however, a member of the group begins to feel the need to explore a past relationship with an abusive parent, which may have had a significant impact upon his or her current attitudes and behaviour, then this would suggest that a referral to a trained counsellor or therapist would be appropriate, alongside (but not instead of) the work you are doing in your group.

### Group exercise

With the help of your tutor or supervisor, as a group think about your current role(s). Where are the boundaries for you and your organisation between generic listening skills and more in-depth work with your service users/clients/patients? Are you clear about how and when you need to refer to other agencies? What are the key agencies in your area who can take these referrals?

## COUNSELLING SKILLS

It should be clear to you now that counselling is a specialist, skilled activity that is probably not part of your own job description. Nor is it appropriate to go into any depth in this book about the communication skills needed for such specialist work. What you will be expected to practise, however, are what are sometimes known as 'counselling skills' or 'active listening skills'. These are the fundamental building blocks for all people-work: they are, if you like, the basic toolkit which is essential for anyone to be able to use effectively if they wish to work with other people. Whether you are a nurse or a social worker; a youth worker or a welfare benefits adviser; a support worker in a homeless unit or someone helping people with drug misuse problems; a doctor's receptionist or a care worker with frail older people with dementia: the core active listening/counselling skills are the essential tools without which you will not be able to do your job effectively.

## FINAL THOUGHTS

There is a vast literature on counselling if you wish to explore it further. The key point for this book, however, is to identify the common skills that every helping professional needs in order to do the job effectively. There are several entries in this book which will help you understand the basic active communication skills that underpin everything you do in your present role.

## REFERENCES AND FURTHER READING

Bach, S. and Grant, A. (2011) *Communication and Interpersonal Skills for Nursing: Transforming Nursing Practice*, 2nd edition. Exeter: Learning Matters.
Feltham, C. and Dryden, W. (1993) *Dictionary of Counselling*. London: Whurr.
Koprowska, J. (2014) *Communication and Interpersonal Skills in Social Work*, 4th edition. Exeter: Learning Matters.
Miller, L. (2012) *Counselling Skills for Social Work*, 2nd edition. London: Sage.
Nelson-Jones, R. (2015) *Theory and Practice of Counselling and Therapy*, 6th edition. London: Sage.

**RELATED CONCEPTS** acceptance; active listening; confidentiality; empathy; establishing a professional relationship; non-verbal communication

**ENGAGING WITH THE PCF** skills and interventions

**ENGAGING WITH THE NMC CODE** prioritise people

## Service user snippet

Joyce (19), social work student:

'I think I really struggled to find my boundaries when working with disturbed young people. I knew it was important to listen to them, and that I wasn't trained to go really deeply into what was hurting them. I didn't want them to feel rejected by sending them off to a therapist, but it was so difficult to find the right words to explain to them what I could and couldn't do.'

# COURT ROOM SKILLS

Without doubt, appearing in court as a professional people-worker can be daunting even to the experienced; to the inexperienced it can be positively frightening. And yet court work can be a significant part of a people-worker's role, especially if your work involves the criminal justice system or family work. You may be called to court because it is your responsibility to prepare a report on someone who has committed an offence, so that the court can come to a fully informed decision about the most appropriate sentence. You may be involved with a family where separation and divorce mean that expert advice needs to be made available to find what is in the best interests of the child(ren) involved. Or you may go to court to offer a character witness for someone you are working with. Whether you attend court regularly or it is more of a 'one off', it is in everyone's best interest that you do as good a job as possible while you are there. Or, as an advice worker, you may have to appear at a tribunal which, although not the same as a court, may make you feel just as nervous.

There is no better way of finding out what a court is like than going to see for yourself.

## Activity

1   Undertake some background reading into the English legal system (or your own country's) so that you can understand its basic principles and procedures. This will also help you understand who does what and where you might fit into the system if called to attend in your professional role. You can also make arrangements to go to your local Magistrates' Court. As a member of the public, you should be allowed to sit in at the back to observe the proceedings. There will be ushers in the entrance area of the court, usually wearing a black gown to make them easily identifiable. Ask them to help you and show you where you can sit. Spend a couple of hours absorbing the atmosphere and getting used to what is happening. That will help you make more sense of the issues we are raising in this discussion.

2   You may, of course, also want to visit a Crown Court that deals with more serious cases, and where a judge will preside. The system is very similar in that you may sit in the public area, and the ushers will help you to find your way around. If you encounter difficulties, write to the clerk to the magistrates and explain why you would like to visit, and you should receive a positive response. You might find it easier to go with another student colleague to share the experience together and reflect on what you have learned.

*(Continued)*

## A point to ponder

Bear in mind also that, as a citizen, you may be called to undertake jury service at some point in your life. This will give you a very clear picture of how the system works, but not everyone is called to do this, and you will have no idea when the summons for jury service letter will drop onto your doormat.

# SOME KEY SKILLS

There are some key skills that are relevant to court work, one of the most important of which is preparation.

## Preparation

General preparation is best undertaken by completing the two introductory activities suggested above. This will help to orientate you to the context of the court and what is expected of you. In your organisation, there should be some more experienced colleagues who can also talk you through what is involved; indeed, you may be able to shadow one of them when they go to court.

Specific preparation becomes necessary when you have a particular reason for going to court. Whether it is a criminal case or a family law matter, it is imperative that you immerse yourself thoroughly in both the detail and the general outline of the case. There may be files you need to read; certainly you will want to meet the people involved and interview them carefully.

## Report writing

If you are preparing a report, there may be other sources of information you need to tap into, and other professionals whose opinions you may need to canvass. Many organisations will have detailed guidelines as to what a report should contain, and you will be required to complete your report succinctly using the agreed headings. There are three skills you need to develop in your report writing.

First, you need to *be brief*. Courts will not want to have to wade through pages and pages of a report: they need information summarised for them succinctly, and this is a really important communication skill you need to develop for this kind of work.

Second, you need to be able to *separate facts from opinions*, and to make this clear in your report. Your professional opinion is certainly valued by the court and will be sought, but you need to separate this out from the facts which need to be stated as part of the background and context.

Third, you need the skill to *make a recommendation* to the court which is legally appropriate, carefully thought through and which draws, where appropriate, upon relevant research and professional knowledge to make it an informed opinion. Bear in mind, though, that you may well be challenged in court over your report, so you need to be confident about what you are saying.

There is a further skill in how you share your report with the person who is the subject of it. They may or may not agree with some of the things you have said. If there are issues of accuracy, then they can help you correct these before the final report is prepared. But often you may be making judgements about them and their behaviour that they may find difficult to accept; they may disagree with the recommendations in the report. This is often the situation in divorce cases where one parent may feel that your recommendations about contact and residence are 'not in their favour'. It is helpful, therefore, to spend enough time with the person to tell them what you are proposing in the report, and to explain why you have come to the conclusions you have. But you can also tell them that, if they disagree, there are avenues open to them to challenge what you are saying. Their solicitor, of course, is the obvious person to do this for them.

Your skills at communicating with the person over your report also need to take into account their ability to read and understand what you have written. It is far too easy to assume that other people can read, so you need to find sensitive ways of checking this out. Some may find a typewritten court report rather daunting to read, and may ask you to read it to them, especially if the language seems too formal. In all cases, however, it is important to give them an opportunity to ask questions about the report, and to be invited to tell you in their own words what the main themes or recommendations are, so that you can be confident that they have understood what has been said about them.

## YOUR DAY IN COURT

There are some useful guidelines for the communication skills you will need in court. The non-verbal communication skills you will use, even before you go into the actual court room, include: dressing appropriately; arriving in good time; making sure you contact the right people who are involved; adopting a professional calm and confident manner (even if the butterflies in your tummy are being hyperactive); and having all the relevant documents and paperwork easily and accessibly available. It is important to seek out the relevant solicitors or barristers to let them know you have arrived, to discuss your report with them and to gain some idea of whether they wish to call you to give evidence. It is helpful to have some advance warning of any issues that they feel need to be expanded on by you, so that you can prepare yourself. You do not always have this luxury but, where possible, do ask them if they think the court will require, or benefit from, additional information from you. Not that you should feel constrained by their views: if you feel strongly that you need to speak up in court, then do ask the appropriate solicitor or barrister to call you to the stand.

When you are called into court by the usher, you will have your designated place. If you have taken the opportunity to go to a court for an observational visit, you will be familiar with what is often called the 'court-room drama and choreography', which you need to understand in order to know where you fit in. This includes everyone standing when the magistrates (or judge) enter; knowing the order in which the various participants make their contributions; and where you need to go in order to give your evidence. You will be asked for your report by the usher who will ensure that the bench (as the magistrates are sometimes referred to) have copies to read.

When called to present your report in a criminal case, you will be guided by the usher to the witness box where your first responsibility is to take the oath to promise 'to tell the truth, the whole truth and nothing but the truth'. There are various options here. The most common of these is to take the Holy Bible in your right hand and to swear your oath. If you belong to other faith communities, there should be other appropriate holy books for you to use instead of the Bible. However, many people feel unhappy about swearing an oath on a holy book; either because they do not believe in what it represents, or as believers they feel it is not right for them to do this. Therefore, it is always possible to make a simple statement or affirmation to the court, promising to tell the truth. Whichever method you choose, the result is the same: you are honour-bound to tell the truth as best you can. To give false information or to seek to deliberately mislead a court are very serious offences, and can be punishable by imprisonment. Your own agency may also take disciplinary action against you if you deliberately seek to mislead the court in any way.

In court proceedings that deal with divorce and family matters, you may find that the whole process is somewhat less formal. You may be called to speak from where you are seated around the table, for example. But the basic rules of behaviour and honesty still apply.

Once in the witness box, you will be asked to confirm your name and your occupation. You may then be asked questions arising from your report. This is the moment when panic may set in; it is also the moment when some basic rules will help you deal with this effectively. These include:

- Take a deep breath and stay looking calm and professional.
- Speak clearly and not too quickly.
- Take your time when answering; it is perfectly acceptable to take a few moments 'thinking time' before you respond to a question.
- State what you know or what you believe, and then stop. If further information is required, you will be asked for it.
- Address your comments directly to the magistrates, and remember to refer to them as 'Your Worship(s)' or, at Crown Court, 'Your Honour'.
- If you are not sure of something, say so. Do not try to cover up your uncertainty with 'off-the-cuff' comments which have not been thought through.
- If you take your file or notes into the witness box and need to refer to them in order to give an answer, first ask the bench if you may refer to them. Take your time in referring to them, but, remember, this is where careful preparation is essential. No one (least of all you) wants to be kept waiting while you struggle to find particular documents in your files.

- Try not to get flustered under cross-examination. Stick to what you have put in the report. By all means, give additional information if you have it, but remember that you probably know more about this case than anyone else in the court, except for the person being dealt with. Answer calmly; give your reasons for your opinion, and let the court decide how much weight to give it. Remember too that it is the job of solicitors or barristers to test out not only the credibility or reliability of the report but also that of the report writer. If they can upset you, or make you flustered, they will have undermined the recommendations you are making. So try to appear calm, even if inside you feel just the opposite.

No one is pretending that this is easy: indeed, confidence comes only with experience and practice. But if you are well prepared and have done your best in presenting the report, you will be a credible witness whom the court will take seriously. Also, take comfort that if the magistrate or judge feels that you are being harassed by a solicitor or barrister, they or the court clerk will often come to your rescue, and admonish the person concerned.

Remember though: it is not personal. People are just doing their jobs, trying to test the truth and doing the best for those whom they represent, just as you are.

## AFTER THE HEARING IS OVER

You may well feel emotionally drained. After all, it is natural to feel that in some ways you and your report have been the ones on trial. You may also feel a bit upset if the court did not follow your recommendation when they decided on their sentence or outcome, but again remember that that is their job and their responsibility. Your task was to furnish them with as much relevant information as possible: their task was to make the decisions.

Whatever the outcome, you will want, if possible, to see the person about whom you prepared the report. They too will most likely be feeling drained, although the outcome will be what affects them most. A post-hearing interview in the cells will feel different from a more relaxed cup of tea in the court canteen, with the person knowing that they can go home. It is, however, important to spend some time going over the outcome with them. In the heat and anxiety of the court room drama, it is not always easy to grasp and retain what is being said; nor are the implications of certain outcomes always fully appreciated. It is good practice, therefore, to talk them through what has been decided, and what must happen next. Ask them to tell you what *they* think has been decided: you can then correct, fine-tune or supplement their response in whatever way you feel is necessary. Often, the solicitor or barrister will also want to talk to them and to you to bring matters to a conclusion, and to make sure that everyone fully understands the outcome.

Before you leave, make sure that any further appointments with you are clearly made and recorded, and remember to say goodbye appropriately.

## Group exercise

With the help of your tutor or supervisor, prepare together a 'mock' court-room scenario that will give you an opportunity to 'get the feel' of being in court and in the witness box. This could be based on a Serious Case Review which highlights issues around giving evidence in court (e.g. *Daniel Pelka, Coventry LSCB, 2/10/13*) or fictitious. Decide who is best placed to play the role of the magistrate and the solicitors who will be asking the questions. Allocate the various professional roles appropriate to the case, and ensure that each of them is called to enter the witness box and present their evidence. This exercise needs careful planning and preparation, but it can be a powerful and valuable learning exercise to help you develop confidence before having to do it 'for real'.

## FINAL THOUGHTS

It is helpful to be able to talk through your time in court with your supervisor, tutor, practice educator or an experienced colleague, to help you offload any anxieties or negative feelings you may have and to bring the whole experience into perspective. If, for example, your recommendation was followed by the court, you may be feeling somewhat elated that you have 'won' and may need to be brought back to earth with a reminder of the work that still has to be done with this person. But primarily, the debriefing will help you identify what went well, and ways in which you could improve your performance on future occasions.

## REFERENCES AND FURTHER READING

Brown, H. and Marriott, A. (2018) *ADR: Principles and Practice*, 4th edition. London: Sweet & Maxwell.

Finch, E. and Fanfinski, S. (2018) *Legal Skills*, 7th edition. Oxford: Oxford University Press.

Partington, M. (2018) *Introduction to the English Legal System*, 2018/2019 edition. Oxford: Oxford University Press.

Seymour, C. and Seymour, R. (2011) *Court Room Skills for Social Workers*, 2nd edition. Exeter: Learning Matters.

**RELATED CONCEPTS** advocacy; anti-discriminatory practice; conflict management; interpreters; non-verbal communication

**ENGAGING WITH THE PCF** skills and interventions; professionalism

**ENGAGING WITH THE NMC CODE** promote professionalism and trust

## Service user snippet

Jason (19), first offence:

'I found going to court first time really scary. My probation officer had explained everything to me and had done a report on me. But then she had to stand up and talk about me in front of everyone else. She was dead cool about it, which was amazing really. She knew her stuff, that's for sure. Good job!'

# DOCUMENTATION, RECORDING AND FORM FILLING

No one would be surprised if your least favourite activity is completing documentation, doing your recording and filling in forms. Whether you are a social worker, a nurse, or are involved in any other people-work profession, the challenges of paperwork can be daunting, time-consuming and at times frustrating, especially if they have to be completed on line. How many times have we been faced with official forms that seem to ask a different set of questions from the ones we feel are most relevant or suitable to the needs of the person we are working with? How often is the requirement to write in plain clear English thwarted by the use of jargon, technical terms or poor grammar and punctuation? And when online, how often does the form refuse to allow us to move to the next section for no apparent reason? We groan inwardly and do our best, but secretly wonder whether the documentation is our servant or our somewhat verbose 'fat controller'!

## Activity

In whatever organisation you are working, ask your supervisor if you can have access to some case records or reports from a few years ago. Read them critically in the light of the principles outlined above. What strikes you from reading these examples of documentation? What might you do differently?

There are, of course, almost as many examples of documentation as there are people to complete them, and it would be impossible to itemise them in this necessarily brief discussion. It is important nonetheless at this point to remind yourself of some key basic principles that underpin the documentation you use.

The first of these is *accountability*. As a professional you are accountable to the agency that employs you, and some aspects of documentation such as record keeping or minute taking at key meetings are an important means of demonstrating that you are working on behalf of the agency and are there to uphold its values and to deliver its services.

You are also accountable to the people whom you seek to help and serve. When you keep records or fill in a report you are trying to represent that person and their needs, especially if the form you are completing on their behalf is going to be sent to another colleague or a different agency in order for decisions to be made. If you do not get it right, then there is little chance of the service user receiving their entitlement. To what extent have you been able to work in partnership?

The second principle is *accuracy*. Is the information you are recording accurate? Have you checked it with the person you are working with so that they agree it is a fair representation of their 'story'? Whether or not you agree with their point of view, have you accurately conveyed it? Are you absolutely clear about why you are making this record and what the principal purpose of it is? If you are not sure, then whatever you write or record is likely to miss its target.

You need also to remember that it may not always be you who is working with this person. Just as you will have consulted case notes or patient records compiled by other colleagues in order to gain a full picture, so too others following you may consult your records and notes to help them decide how most effectively to help or to intervene. Accuracy is really important: you may not be there to explain to another colleague what you really meant!

*Honesty* is another important principle. Your professional integrity is challenged with every sentence you write, and with every judgement you make. You will have your prejudices just like everyone else: how do you ensure that these do not cloud your judgement? Are you able to separate facts from opinions? We talk about this in the entry on court-room skills and report writing, but it applies right across the board. To what extent is the language you use capable of misinterpretation? For example, if you refer to someone as being 'difficult', is this saying more about you than it is about them? How do you handle situations where your personal or professional values are at odds with those of the person you are writing a report on?

*Clarity* is also crucial. You need to be clear about the 'audience' you are addressing. If what you are recording is strictly 'in house', then you may be able to use professional jargon or shorthand or medical terminology that is only meaningful to a fellow professional. But if you are writing for a wider audience, then finding the appropriate language and terminology that conveys your meaning with absolute clarity is an essential skill. Writing in clear English is not as easy as some people think!

*Security*. You also need to be aware of who will have access to your documentation. The heightened awareness of data protection issues means that you need to consider issues of confidentiality, written permission for access to, or sharing with others, the information you are documenting, and where the information will be securely stored. This is both a personal as well as an organisational issue. Are you allowed to store confidential information on your personal computer, for example? What guarantees are there that your system won't be hacked into? And how many examples can you think of where someone has had their car broken into and confidential information stolen, or they have lost memory sticks or disks with sensitive data stored on them? Security of information is an essential principle to safeguard.

## Group exercise

With the help of your tutor or supervisor, read the Coventry Safeguarding Children Board's Serious Case Review for Baby F (Agnew, 2016) where 'poor-quality and inconsistent record keeping' were highlighted. Bring your thoughts and reactions to your group discussion with your tutor or supervisor to help you all identify the key learning points emerging for you.

## FINAL THOUGHTS

The principles outlined above underpin all the documentation, report writing, minute taking and form filling that you will undertake in your professional role. The more you understand these principles, the more you will appreciate the importance of getting it right; of refusing to be 'slapdash' in completing your written tasks, and of remembering that you are the front line of the agency you represent whenever you are working with an individual or family. You never stop being accountable.

## REFERENCES AND FURTHER READING

Agnew, D. (2016) *Coventry Safeguarding Children Board Serious Case Review: Baby F.* Coventry: CSCB. Available at file:///C:/Users/Solveig/Downloads/Child_F__Serious_Case_Review__Overview_Report_.pdf (accessed 20/10/19).

Bogg, D. (2016) *Report Writing* (Social work pocket book). Maidenhead: Open University Press.

Hopkins, G. (1998) *Plain English for Social Services: A Guide to Better Communication.* Lyme Regis: Russell House.

Thompson, N. (2018) *Effective Communication: A Guide for the People Professions*, 3rd edition. Basingstoke: Palgrave Macmillan.

Trevithick, P. (2012) *Social Work Skills and Knowledge: A Practice Handbook*, 3rd edition. Maidenhead: Open University Press.

Web resource

Nursing & Midwifery Council, Record keeping guidance: www.nmc.org/standards/code/record-keeping (accessed 11/09/2019)

**RELATED CONCEPTS** confidentiality; court-room skills (report writing); establishing a professional relationship

**ENGAGING WITH THE PCF** skills and interventions; contexts and organisations; professionalism

**ENGAGING WITH THE NMC CODE** promote professionalism and trust

---

Service user snippet

Jason (21):

'When I got to court like … I thought me social worker were sound like – but when me solicitor read the report on me I freaked out – it were a pack of lies.'

# ECOMAPS

Ecomaps are similar to genograms in that they are pictorial representations of relationships between people, which you can use both as an aid to recording and interpreting information, and also as a direct tool in your work with people.

## BUILDING BLOCK 1

The basic building block for an ecomap is an empty circle drawn on a piece of paper, and repeated for as many times as there are people in the relationship network you are seeking to explore and understand. The easiest way is to draw a circle to represent the person with whom you are currently working, and then to think about the other people in that person's life whom they (or you) wish to include in the picture. The crucial idea of the ecomap is that the distance between the central circle/person and other characters is an important indicator. This could be used simply to represent geographical distance between people, so that family members are placed closest to the central character, and people who live at a distance are situated towards the edge of your page. Or the distances on the page could represent the importance of the people in the central character's life, whereby those most important are situated closest to the centre. People who matter less will be placed out towards the margins, even if they happen to live in the same household. In other words, with this use of an ecomap, the closer each person is emotionally to the central character, the nearer they are located to the central circle. By contrast, people who are of less significance or importance are located some way out on the edge of the paper. For example, in Figure 2, the ecomap uses physical closeness as the key, but in Figure 3 it is emotional closeness that is the driver.

The ecomap in Figure 2 suggests that A is living at home with his parents P and M, and that there are three friends, X, Y and Z, who are important in A's life – they could be friends at school, perhaps.

The ecomap in Figure 3 suggests that the people who are emotionally closest to A in the centre are X, Y and Z, but that crucially P, A's father, although he lives at home with the family, is seen to be distant, and is perceived by A to have a less important influence on A's life.

## BUILDING BLOCK 2

Into these various circles, you can, if you wish or think it is important, write some key information, such as the names, ages or attributes of each person. If you were working with a young person who was struggling with issues to do with peer pressure, for example, it might be very important to know the ages and characteristics of each of the players who appear on the ecomap, and how these impact upon the person you are working with. The ecomap shown in Figure 3 would also be enhanced by knowing how old A was – there may be different lessons and implications to be drawn if A was 8, 18 or 28, for example.

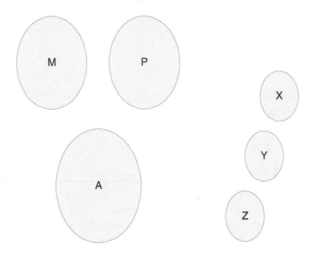

**Figure 2**   Physical closeness

*Source*: © Tony Jones. Reproduced with permission.

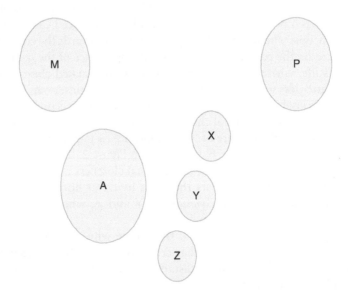

**Figure 3**   Emotional closeness

*Source*: © Tony Jones. Reproduced with permission.

## BUILDING BLOCK 3

In some ways, the fun now starts, because at this stage it is possible to use some different symbols to represent the quality of the relationships between the key players.

As with the interpretative use of genograms, with ecomaps you can use a jagged zig-zaggy line between two people to represent friction, aggression and hostility between them. By contrast, thick strong continuous lines can be used to represent strong relationships between A and those who are most important in A's life, for whatever reason. A thinner line would suggest that the relationship is still important but of lesser significance than the relationship portrayed by the thick line. A dotted line would imply that there is an element of 'take it or leave it' about your relationship to that person.

These observations demonstrate how simple and straightforward the use of ecomaps can be, but also how effectively in just a simple picture a very powerful story can be depicted.

## Activity

### Stage 1

This is probably a good point at which to pause and invite you to 'have a go' for yourself to see how an ecomap works. As with any tool you select to enhance your practice with people, you need to be confident about why you are using it and what benefits it can bring to your work, and also what risks you may run if you do decide to use it directly with people.

As a starter, draw an ecomap of your life and your relationships using geographical distance as the driver. This means that you will draw a circle for each person who lives with you in the same household in close proximity to the circle you have drawn to represent yourself. Other people who are important to you, but who live away from you, can be placed on your ecomap at appropriate distances from you.

When you have completed the location of all the people you wish to include, then think about your actual relationship with them, and use a combination of strong lines, weak lines, dotted lines and jagged lines to represent how you feel about your relationship with them.

### Stage 2

This time, use the idea of emotional significance as the driver for your ecomap. This means that with your own circle again centrally placed on the page, you draw circles close to you representing the people who mean the most to you, and place out towards the edges of the paper those who matter the least to you, depending upon how distant you feel from them emotionally. Put names in each circle so that they become real to you for this exercise.

As before, it is again useful to draw in the relationship lines on the ecomap to indicate clearly which relationships are most nurturing and which are most stressful.

## Group exercise

With the help of your tutor or supervisor, think about the network of colleagues or agencies with whom you are involved on a daily basis. Ecomaps can help you evaluate and better understand the complex relationships between colleagues, agencies and organisations, both for their general level of collaboration and also in specific instances where several agencies are working together with a particular individual or family. Choose an example from your own practice and, with a group of colleagues, draw an ecomap that best reflects the level of collaborative working between you.

## A NOTE OF CAUTION

It will have become clear to you in completing these activities that this deceptively easy tool can be immensely powerful. If you take the issues that it raises seriously, especially in relation to stressful relationships, you can very quickly find yourself in touch with some powerful, even disturbing feelings. This should be a warning to you, therefore, to handle such tools with care, and to regard them as just that: powerful communication tools to be used creatively, but with caution. It is one thing to use this tool as a way of recording information after an interview and to reflect on the issues that are raised. It is another matter when you begin to use ecomaps in direct work with people. If, therefore, you find yourself getting into difficult territory, it is important to use the same degree of sensitivity as always. The ecomap may well have triggered off some powerful feelings that need to be acknowledged. Sometimes you will need to have the courage to put the tool to one side, if need be, and to work with the person in whatever way seems best. There is no particular merit in pressing on in a mechanistic way just to gather information at a surface level, and certainly no justification for pressing on into territory which the person you are working with would find too distressing to handle.

## FINGERS ON THE BUTTONS

So far, we have talked about how you can use a pen and paper or flip chart and marker pen to draw an ecomap, and we have seen how effective and powerful this can be. There is another variation that deserves mention, not least because it can be used with young people and with people who have mild communication difficulties. This variation uses a tin of buttons instead of pen and paper.

You need to have a fairly large tin with a variety of shapes, colours and sizes of buttons. This approach is very much for direct work with people, and has the merit of being interactive. In essence, it provides a dynamic ecomap.

After an appropriate introduction as to why this tool is being used, the person with whom you are working is invited to choose a button from the tin that best represents who they are. They put this in the middle of the table – perhaps with an invitation from you to say why that particular button appeals to them and why they have chosen it. Then you ask them to think about people who are important in that person's life, and to choose a button to represent each of them in turn. Then invite them to place that button somewhere on the table to present how close they feel to that person. After a while, you will end up with several different buttons on the table representing the various people in that person's life. You then have the opportunity to ask about each of them (or you could do this as each button is placed in position).

Again, this can be very powerful as the picture unfolds, and sometimes strong feelings are evoked, especially if you move a particular button closer, or further away, from the central button and explore how that would feel to the person with whom you are working.

## FINAL THOUGHTS

As with many tools which can be used to enhance communication skills, ecomaps can be powerful visual representations of complex and at times distressing realities about people's relationships. They can also represent strengths, support systems and networks, and ways in which people's resilience can be enhanced. It is up to you as a worker to decide how to use such tools most effectively, and what themes and issues you feel need to be explored further.

But there is also a warning to be sounded here: however much you may feel you wish to be in charge, it is important to stress that ecomaps are powerful *precisely because* they put the person with whom you are working into the driving seat. Ecomaps can be excellent tools for real partnership working. It will be up to you, therefore, to listen attentively, so that what you begin to really focus on is what is important to that person, and not what you find easiest to handle.

## REFERENCES AND FURTHER READING

Coulshed, V. and Orme, J. (2012) *Social Work Practice*, 5th edition. Basingstoke: Palgrave Macmillan.
Parker, J.R. and Bradley, G. (2014) *Social Work Practice: Assessment, Planning, Intervention and Review*, 4th edition. Exeter: Learning Matters.

Web resource

SmartDraw, drawing tool – www.smartdraw.com (accessed 15/10/19)

**RELATED CONCEPTS** assessment; empowerment; genograms

**ENGAGING WITH THE PCF** contexts and organisations; interprofessional collaboration; skills and interventions

**ENGAGING WITH THE NMC CODE** practise effectively; promote professionalism and trust

---

### Service user snippet

Malcolm (10), young person in care:

'I liked using the buttons to draw my map of my family and friends ... I was a bit puzzled at first but then it was fun and I could talk to the buttons instead of to Lucy [my social worker].'

# EMOTIONAL INTELLIGENCE (EI)

Emotional intelligence (EI) is of fundamental importance to people-work simply because we work with people, who all have emotions! This is such an obvious thing to say, but we ignore it at our peril if we want to deliver sensitive best practice.

EI builds on the very familiar concept of our intelligence quotient (IQ), for which various psychological and psychometric tests and measures are available to assess and measure our level of intelligence. IQ testing is not an exact science, although it does provide some useful benchmarks. But, more importantly, it does not tell the whole story of who we are, what our potential is, how successful we can become, what our hopes and fears may be or how we handle ourselves and others when we are caught up in an emotionally charged situation. Dealing with emotionally charged situations, however, is part and parcel of people-work, and we owe it to ourselves and to those with whom we work to be able to handle this aspect of our work as confidently as possible.

(*Note*: Because IQ is such a familiar concept, Goleman (1996, 1998) and others (e.g. Howe, 2008; Held, 2009) have built up a 'family' or hierarchy of similar 'Q's and have developed the notions of emotional and spiritual intelligence, which are often known as EQ and SQ, although strictly speaking the use of 'Q' meaning 'quotient', thereby suggesting scientific measurable outcomes, is not appropriate for EQ and SQ.)

---

## Activity

Think for a moment about the work you do. Can you recall a recent situation where emotions ran high? How did you react and respond?

---

This Activity is an important place to begin this discussion because the emotional dimension of people-work is so central. Whether you are a nurse caring for someone who has just received some bad news about their health; a social worker involved in removing a child into care; safeguarding a vulnerable adult or engaging with a person with mental health difficulties; a youth worker trying to calm down a distressed and aggressive young person, in all these situations and many more, emotions can run high, and you need to be able to deal with them effectively.

But it is not just emotions in other people. You can just as easily allow your own emotions to influence how you treat other people. If, for example, you had a blazing argument with your partner before leaving for work; if you are really worried about having sent your child to nursery or school when they were not feeling very well; if you have serious worries about your health or the stability of your relationship at home; if you feel that you are not being properly supported at work and are made to feel undervalued or exploited, in all these situations and many more, you risk letting your emotions influence, or even take over, how you react to other people.

People-work, therefore, can sometimes be intensely emotional, and EI is all about helping you to recognise the emotional dimension of your work and to develop and maintain the skills you need to handle these issues in a mature, professional and sensitive manner.

EI/EQ is popularly linked with the work of Daniel Goleman (1996, 1998, 2000), whose very accessible writings suggest that it is a high level of EI/EQ, rather than intellectual brilliance, that helps people to achieve success, especially (we would suggest) in the helping professions. Goleman was particularly interested in the contribution that EI/EQ can make to successful leadership and management in industry and business, and it is interesting to see how these ideas have become influential in major multinational companies and government departments, including the NHS (NHS Institute for Innovation and Improvement, 2006). Goleman (1998: 317) defined EI as a 'capacity for recognising our own and others' feelings, for motivating ourselves, and for managing our emotions, both within ourselves and in our relationships.' He then identified five key elements of EI/EQ: self-awareness, self-regulation, motivation, empathy and social skills.

Important though these aspects of EI are to all leaders and managers, they are particularly important within people-work at all levels in an organisation. Whatever your role in your organisation, therefore, you need to develop strong and confident EI in order to do your work effectively and to a high standard.

Thompson (2012) discusses a helpful acronym – *SARAH* – to help you when you encounter an emotionally fraught situation. SARAH provides practical guidance for EI/EQ as follows:

*S = Stop talking:* As a people-worker, you need to be able to listen carefully and attentively, and to resist the urge to talk the other person down.

*A = Actively listen:* If you can be attentive, using good non-verbal communication, and give the other person who is emotionally upset time to get things off their chest, you will have made a good start. Show the other person that you really do care about them and how they are feeling. What some people need, in effect, is a good listening to!

*R = Reflect content or feeling:* This is a key skill in your active listening. From time to time, it is helpful to mirror back to the person who is upset some of the feelings and words they are using. This shows you are hearing what they are saying and feeling; it gives them an opportunity to respond, especially if they feel you have not fully grasped what they are saying or feeling.

*A = A*ct with empathy: This is easier said than done, of course. It involves skill in helping the other person feel that you recognise and acknowledge what they are feeling; that you are taking the time to walk alongside them on their particularly painful journey. The skill comes in making sure that you do not become so caught up in how they are feeling that you lose your professional balance and become part of their problem.

*H = H*andle objections: You won't always get it right and, from time to time, the person you are listening to may object to something you or someone else has said or done, or complain in some way. It is important not to ignore such objections, but to acknowledge them as honestly and as fully as you can. This will show that whatever is thrown at you (verbally, that is – if you are afraid of imminent physical violence, you must protect yourself and leave), you have heard it and will do your best to handle it. If you are seen to weather some of the emotional storm with the other person, you are much more likely to earn their respect and to be able to work with them more effectively.

## Group exercise

With the help of your tutor or supervisor, work together as a group to explore how the SARAH approach can help you develop your EI. Identify some scenarios and then work in pairs to practise using SARAH, spending no more than 10 minutes on each one. Afterwards, share your reactions and give feedback. What went well? What were the challenges using this approach?

Don't be disheartened if you find this exercise challenging. EI is sensitive and may take time for some people to develop confidence. Group exercises in a safe environment with tutor and supervisor support are excellent ways of developing this crucial attribute in your personal and professional approach to people.

### Implications for leadership

Everything we have said so far applies to any and every people-worker, but it has a particular resonance with colleagues who occupy a leadership role. It can be argued that EI/EQ is even more important for leaders because they are not only responsible for themselves; they are also responsible for the wellbeing and flourishing of those committed to their care and management.

The pressures upon leaders and managers in so many organisations are ever increasing. Achieving targets; allocating increasing caseloads; coping with and planning for change; delivering more with fewer resources: these everyday complaints by leaders and managers are all too common. There is therefore a strong temptation in such situations to withdraw into a managerial shell; to deal with issues in a mechanistic way and to ignore the human and emotional turmoil that may be bubbling below the surface. The bullying leader is often a scared leader, afraid of the emotional maelstrom that threatens to boil over.

And yet to ignore this crucial aspect of leadership is a dereliction of duty. People are people, whether they are service users, nurses, workers, leaders or managers, and the emotional aspects of who they are, what they are doing and how they are doing it are all important. The chances are that, if emotional aspects are recognised and valued, there will be a better job done all round; if they are ignored, then distress and underperformance will ensue.

Good and effective managers therefore will not only acknowledge and respect their own emotions, but will find time and opportunity to recognise these aspects of their team members' professional, and at times, personal lives. Purposeful supervision plays an important role in this; and so does the day-to-day contact and encouragement that a leader can bring to team dynamics.

Leadership and management will still be stressful; organisational expectations, which are sometimes unrealistic and oppressive, will take their toll, and even the strongest can falter or crack under the pressure. All organisations have a duty of care to all their employees at every level. But EI/EQ plays a crucial role in helping leaders and managers draw the best out of their team as well as enhancing their own resilience and wellbeing.

## EI and leadership – nursing perspectives

EI plays a significant part in effective communication. By developing the skills to engage in conversations with others you can learn when, as a nurse, to contribute to the conversation and when to step away. By understanding and controlling your own emotions, you can recognise the emotions of others. As a nurse you will often work in emotionally challenging situations, and by developing EI you can support others whilst reducing your stress levels.

There are many situations as a nurse when you will need to manage your emotions, for example, in developing professional relationships, managing conflict, breaking bad news or providing leadership. Leadership is a vital component of contemporary nursing practice and features strongly in the *Standards for Pre-registration Nursing Programmes* (NMC, 2018a), *Future Nurse: Standards of Proficiency for Registered Nurses* (NMC, 2018b) and the *The Code: Professional Standards of Practice* (NMC, 2018c). The NMC Code provides clear guidance on the leadership skills that nurses must possess and demonstrate:

> Provide leadership to make sure people's wellbeing is protected and to improve their experience of the health and care system,

and sets out a range of standards that all nurses must adhere to and leadership behaviours that must be demonstrated.

EI is a key feature of nursing and nursing leadership. By developing your EI and leadership skills, you can promote best practice and protect the people in your care.

## NHS Leadership Academy

There is now the NHS Leadership Academy, which supports the development of leaders in the NHS. They have developed a new national leadership development framework (see National Improvement and Leadership Development Board, 2016).

## FINAL THOUGHTS

It is important to return to the issue of your own emotions. Part of your professional responsibility is to be sufficiently self-aware so that you do not allow your own emotional *baggage* to get in the way of the work you are doing. From time to time, however, you will need help and support to do this, and it is up to you to seek out the most appropriate person. There will be occasions when you have a professional duty to notify your manager about your situation so that appropriate steps can be taken, not just to support you but also to ensure that best practice can be maintained.

## REFERENCES AND FURTHER READING

Goleman, D. (1996) *Emotional Intelligence: Why It Can Matter More than IQ*. London: Bloomsbury Publishing.

Goleman, D. (1998) *Working with Emotional Intelligence*. London: Bloomsbury.

Goleman, D. (2000) 'Leadership that gets results', *Harvard Business Review*, 7 (2): 78–90.

Held, S. (2009) 'Emotional intelligence, emotion and collaborative leadership', Chapter 7 in J. McKimm and K. Phillips (eds), *Leadership and Management in Integrated Services*. Exeter: Learning Matters.

Howe, D. (2008) *The Emotionally Intelligent Social Worker*. Basingstoke: Palgrave Macmillan.

NHS Institute for Innovation and Improvement (2006) *Leadership Qualities Framework*. Available at www.nhsleadershipqualities.nhs.uk (accessed 28/12/16).

National Improvement and Leadership Development Board (2016) 'Developing People – Improving Care: a national framework for action on improvement and leadership development in NHS-funded services'. Available at https://improvement.nhs.uk/documents/542/Developing_People-Improving_Care-010216.pdf (accessed 20/10/19).

Nursing & Midwifery Council (NMC) (2018a) *Realising Professionalism – Part 3: Standards for Pre-registration Nursing Programmes*. London: NMC.

Nursing & Midwifery Council (NMC) (2018b) *Future Nurse: Standards of Proficiency for Registered Nurses*. London: NMC.

Nursing & Midwifery Council (NMC) (2018c) *The Code: Professional Standards of Practice and Behaviour for Nurses, Midwives and Nursing Associates*. London: NMC.

Thompson, N. (2012) *The People Solutions Sourcebook*, 2nd edition. Basingstoke: Palgrave Macmillan.

**RELATED CONCEPTS** active listening; breaking bad news; feedback; non-verbal communication; spirituality

**ENGAGING WITH THE PCF** skills and intervention; professional leadership; professionalism; values and ethics

**ENGAGING WITH THE NMC CODE** prioritise people

E

## Service user snippet

Aisha (23), resident in a women's refuge:

'I don't care how much these workers know … if they can't show me some warmth and some honest-to-goodness care for me, then forget it!'

# EMPATHY

Within a wide range of people-work, 'empathy' is a key buzzword, which characterises a high-quality relationship between the worker and the person being listened to or helped. Several metaphors have been used to try to capture the essence of empathy, one of the most popular being that of 'wearing another person's shoes'. The idea behind this is a simple one: empathy is about trying to see the world from the other person's point of view; to get inside how the other person really feels, so that you can begin to see things through their eyes. Only then will that person feel that they have been accepted and fully listened to. Rogers (1957: 99) described empathy as the ability 'to sense the client's private world as if it were your own, but without ever losing the "as if" quality – this is empathy.'

A distinction is sometimes drawn between sympathy and empathy. We can all feel sympathy towards someone who is going through a difficult time, and we express this by saying how sorry we are, and offering to do anything we can to help. Sympathy is an emotion or feeling that is generated within us by the misfortune of others, and in that sense is part of what it means to be genuinely and fully human. The world would be a poorer place if we were not moved by tragedy and misfortune to offer a variety of responses to others. Indeed, much charitable work, on an individual and corporate level, is a channelling of these sympathetic responses in practical, as well as emotional, ways.

Empathy builds upon this sympathetic streak within us, but seeks to develop a far more interactive relationship with the other person. It is, of course, impossible to fully 'get inside another person's skin' (another metaphor sometimes used), but the attempt to do so is hugely important within a professional relationship. It is only when the other person begins to feel that you really *do* understand 'where they are coming from', and can glimpse the world from their point of view, that they will begin to feel accepted and encouraged to begin a journey towards whatever changes in their lives are necessary.

It is in this sense that empathy can be regarded as a communication skill that needs to be recognised, practised and developed. Perhaps it is not a skill in the strict sense of the word; maybe it says more about the outcome of other communication skills being used effectively. Nevertheless, it is an outcome that a skilled helper can achieve within a professional relationship, without leaving it to chance.

Koprowska (2014: 47) captures the challenge of empathic listening when she talks about 'empathic attunement', which carries the notion of someone trying to tune into a particular radio or television wavelength to listen to a particular programme. The signals are out there, but it needs some careful and sensitive work on the part of the person adjusting the tuner to 'home in' on the signal so that it is loud and clear. The skill lies in that careful and sensitive adjustment to hear the other person's programme with maximum clarity.

The development of empathic skills is an issue that has taxed trainers and educators alike. Controlled outcome studies by Nerdrum and Lundquist (1995) and

Nerdrum (1997) explored the effectiveness of communication skills training in increasing students' capacity to be empathetic. There was sufficient evidence from these studies to argue for these skills to be included in basic communication skills training courses, in spite of other studies which were more sceptical (e.g. Barber, 1988). There is also a wider concern about how students are able to transfer the skills gained in the training context into their eventual professional practice (Dickson and Bamford, 1995). Although this remains a largely under-researched issue, the implications from these findings are clear: there is no automatic achievement of empathetic attunement, and workers need to put every effort into achieving this goal with those with whom they are professionally engaged.

The following suggestions and examples may help you to develop your skills in this area. They are based on guidelines that have been drawn up by tutors at the University of Manchester (unpublished) involved in training medical students in communication skills, but are applicable to a wide range of people-workers. They are not foolproof, and must always be used with sensitivity, but if used well, they can help you build up an empathic rapport with the person with whom you are working.

- *Acknowledge verbal cues*: 'You've just told me how sad/angry/upset you feel when ...'
- *Acknowledge non-verbal cues*: 'You seem to me to be very tense/angry/upset.'
- *Use tentative questions*: 'I'm wondering whether you feel this way because of ...'
- *Use self-disclosure, where appropriate*: 'I think that if that were me, I would feel very shocked/upset by what you have just described to me.'
- *Use your imagination*: 'I imagine you must have felt very ...'
- *Consider using gentle touch*: Reaching out gently to touch the person's hand, arm or shoulder can sometimes be a powerful expression of empathic attunement, but obviously it needs to be carefully considered, especially across gender or cultural boundaries. If in doubt, it is better not to risk it, but you will be surprised at how even a slight movement of the hand towards the other person can be equally effective.
- *Use mirroring*: Adjust your tone of voice, posture and gestures to mirror those of the other person. This can convey a strong rapport, but can also be rather off-putting if done mechanistically. Sometimes, however, if the other person is sitting in a very enclosed posture with arms folded and so on, you can begin by mirroring that posture, and slowly but deliberately open up your own posture to encourage them to follow.

## Activity

To complete this Activity, you will need to have someone with whom you can discuss some examples from your work, and who can help you explore your effectiveness at developing empathy. Your supervisor, line manager or practice educator should be able to help, but it is important that you can trust them to work with you at a fairly deep level. In a word, you need to be confident that *they* can establish an empathic relationship with *you*.

## Group exercise

With the help of your tutor or supervisor, identify some scenarios where empathy will be particularly important. For example, supporting parents with a child who has a life-limiting condition, or being engaged in end-of-life care. Consider ways of 'tuning in' to the person in the scenario, perhaps using the unpublished Manchester University guidelines mentioned above (p. 115). Then, working in pairs, practise for a few minutes developing appropriate questions and comments. Give feedback afterwards to help develop your confidence.

Don't be disheartened if this is difficult – it is! But if in this safe environment with the help of your tutor or supervisor you can develop the ability to respond with warmth and empathy, the people you work with will really appreciate it.

### Empathy: dealing with upset people

In professional working roles, there can often – and almost inevitably – be occasions when you are working with service users or patients who may not agree with some of the decisions which you seek to encourage or make regarding their individual case, or with the information you are communicating to them. However much you may succeed in empathising, their reaction towards you may at times be disconcerting.

Realistically, this can sometimes lead to people exhibiting abusive, intimidating, aggressive or threatening behaviour towards you – which can make you feel naturally anxious and worried for your safety. These types of situations can also lead to you doubting your own decision making. It is important to recognise that part of the unconscious reasoning for service users or patients behaving in this way may be due to the power they feel you hold as a professional.

It is essential that the way you respond does not fuel a situation further – so if someone is shouting at you, make sure that you respond with a calm tone of voice and manner. Ensure that your body language is positive and controlled, and avoid responding with equally threatening or abusive behaviour. Even if you do feel threatened, try not to show it.

If a service user or patient can see that you are feeling scared and anxious, they may feel that they 'have the upper hand'. Whilst empowerment is a skill which we try to encourage in service users, it is not helpful if the 'empowered' individual then were to act inappropriately, perhaps thereby putting you as a worker at risk.

Stress, crisis and coping are further key aspects to consider. People may view stress differently, as:

- a threat – response will be 'fight or flight';
- a challenge – response will be to focus on learning and development;
- an opportunity – response will be positive and optimistic with an openness to new experiences.

Coping is defined as the response we bring to the problem situation (which will differ depending on the way that stress is defined). The ways we handle the problem are referred to as 'coping mechanisms'. The mechanisms we draw on will depend on:

- our personality;
- the way we define the 'problem';
- the way we perceive stress;
- the resources we have;
- our repertoire (the patterns of behaviour we have learnt).

However, it may simply be that the service user or patient does not recognise or understand what you are saying to them, and why. If on further exploration this is the case, then time must be taken to undertake discussion with them. Good empathic listening skills are essential so that a full understanding of the reasons for their 'angst' is fully understood. This will also demonstrate your genuine interest in the service user, to enable your professional relationship to remain intact.

Sometimes in medical contexts it is particularly difficult fully to understand what is being explained, and not every doctor has the ability to ensure that the patient has grasped the full picture, especially if they have no one with them to support them. In such situations it might well fall to the nurse, or the social worker, to spend time ensuring that the patient is not grappling with unanswered questions. It can be helpful to 'chunk and check': in other words, to go through the issues step by step and ensure at each point that everyone fully understands. It may be beneficial for the communication to be 'stripped back' to the bare essentials: that is, what you are trying to achieve, why you are trying to achieve it, and the advantages in doing so. Further explanation could quite simply be the key to calming a situation down and ensuring that the service user continues to work with you. Also, where possible, negotiation skills can be used to encourage working together.

Checking understanding can be particularly important for people with learning disabilities, older people and those with mental health issues who may also lack mental capacity, for example. Some people may 'talk the talk' but still not fully understand. The needs of the individual must be held at the forefront to ensure the best outcomes are achieved. Sometimes you may need to involve an advocate to ensure that a full understanding is achieved.

It must also be noted that professional workers may occasionally be subjected to physical abuse and/or aggression by service users or patients. If you encounter any behaviour where you feel that your safety may be compromised, you must try to leave immediately, call for support from colleagues, or if appropriate the relevant emergency services. A reflective supervision would be beneficial following any such incident. You too can become upset, and your resilience can be undermined, so it is important that you seek appropriate support. Empathy is an essential attribute for any people-worker. It facilitates the helping process and reflects the values of openness and respect. It can minimise risk and enable empowerment. But it cannot remove all risks, and you need always to keep yourself safe.

## FINAL THOUGHTS

Getting inside someone else's world view is also one of the main themes of the contemporary debate about spirituality, with its interest in 'what makes people tick', how they view the world and what gives them meaning and purpose in their lives. As we engage with people at this deeper level of empathic attunement, we may begin to understand the deeper relevance of this theme of spirituality to our work with other people.

## REFERENCES AND FURTHER READING

Barber, J. (1988) 'Are microskills worth teaching?', *Journal of Social Work Education*, Winter (1): 3–12.

Dickson, D. and Bamford, D. (1995) 'Improving the interpersonal skills of social work students: the problem of transfer of training and what to do about it', *British Journal of Social Work*, 25 (1): 85–105.

Egan, G. (2013) *The Skilled Helper*, 10th international edition. Belmont CA: Brooks/Cole.

Koprowska, J. (2014) *Communication and Interpersonal Skills in Social Work*, 4th edition. Exeter: Learning Matters.

Nelson-Jones, R. (2014) *Theory and Practice of Counselling and Therapy*, 6th edition. London: Sage.

Nerdrum, P. (1997) 'Maintenance of the effect of training in communication skills: a controlled follow-up study of level of communicated empathy', *British Journal of Social Work*, 27 (5): 705–22.

Nerdrum, P. and Lundquist, K. (1995) 'Does participation in communication skills training increase student levels of communicated empathy? A controlled outcome study', *Journal of Teaching in Social Work*, 12 (1–2): 139–57.

Rogers, C.R. (1957) 'The necessary and sufficient conditions of therapeutic personality change', *Journal of Consulting Psychology*, 21 (2): 95–103.

Trevithick, P. (2012) *Social Work Skills: A Practice Handbook*, 3rd edition. Maidenhead: Open University Press. See pp. 194–6.

**RELATED CONCEPTS** active listening; anti-discriminatory practice; assertiveness; conflict management; emotional intelligence; establishing a professional relationship; non-verbal communication; reflective practice; resilience; spirituality; supervision; values and ethics

**ENGAGING WITH THE PCF** critical reflection and analysis; professionalism; skills and interventions; values and ethics

**ENGAGING WITH THE NMC CODE** prioritise people; practise effectively

### Service user snippet

Josh (23), social work student:

'Everyone talks about empathy and makes it sound so easy and straightforward … but it isn't – it's really hard work and I don't think it happens all that often if I'm honest – which doesn't mean we should stop trying – just try harder, I suppose.'

# EMPOWERMENT, RESILIENCE AND A STRENGTHS PERSPECTIVE

We are dealing here with a clutch of interrelated concepts – all of which are effectively dealt with at length in a range of professional literature, but which, from a communication skills perspective, can usefully be viewed together. They all deal with the impact that you hope your intervention skills will have on the people with whom you are working: from feeling perhaps disempowered, helpless and overwhelmed, you hope that they will emerge at the end of the helping process much better able and equipped to cope, feeling much more in control of their lives, and in touch with the powers of resilience and inner strengths, of which, under the pressures of their problems, they had temporarily lost sight.

There is a clear overlap of values and skills here. You have a responsibility as a people-worker to examine your value base, and how this informs your view of the people who come to you for help. You can be sure that how you feel about other people will come across in your non-verbal communication. If, for example, you view your service users, clients or patients as people without hope, vision or 'moral fibre', or as 'inadequate', 'incapable', 'irresponsible', 'misfits', 'deviants' or 'scroungers', it will be almost impossible to disguise these value judgements in the way in which you deal with them. People will quickly get the message about how you *really* regard them.

The question has then to be asked: is this how you would like to be treated if the tables were turned? The likelihood is that you would hate to be treated or regarded in such a way. You would regard it as being insulting, degrading and demeaning. At this point, it will dawn on you how easy it is to fall prey to the trap of professional pride, in which the world falls into two groups: the helpers and the helped. You, the helper, are basically OK, you are competent and deserving of respect; on the other hand, those who need to be helped are somehow second-class citizens to be pitied; they may be offered a helping hand, but somehow they are of less worth.

This stark juxtaposition of viewpoints is intended to highlight the power of value judgements, and the ways in which they can obstruct best anti-discriminatory practice. It is also intended to reveal the falseness of such an approach. Unless you work from a value base that accords dignity and respect to each and every other human being, no matter what their circumstances, you are running the risk of developing this two-tier mentality which can be so destructive of good people-work.

It will be quite different, of course, if your value base reflects an alternative approach. If you view other people as having the capacity for good as well as evil; as having latent strengths as well as inherent weaknesses; as having the potential for taking control over their lives even in the most difficult of circumstances, then this approach will communicate itself in both subtle and direct ways in how you work with people. At a very profound level, this is at the heart of all communication skills in people-work.

How you go about achieving this is the big challenge, although by now it should be clear that the first, and biggest, step is clarifying your own mind map and how you regard those who come to you for help. From the basic stance of according dignity, respect and acceptance to each person, there flows a set of communication skills that you will need to cultivate and develop. These include acceptance, explaining, encouraging, asking and task sharing.

## ACCEPTANCE

The basic communication skill of demonstrating to another person that you accept them, 'warts and all', is a fundamental starting point for all empowerment.

## EXPLAINING

'Explaining' is a relatively simple skill to use, and people-workers sometimes overlook how helpful and liberating it can be for people to be offered explanations. Sometimes, when we are feeling overwhelmed, we can't see things clearly: we talk about 'not being able to see the wood for the trees', and what we often need is for someone to explain things to us. Classic examples of this are official communications from people in authority. It does not seem to matter that every effort has been made by them to write to us in clear, plain English; in the heat of the moment, people can panic and assume the worst. Sometimes, therefore, your role is to read such communications carefully, and to explain what is being said 'in words of one syllable'. On occasion, the letter may well make people feel that the worst is imminent – that they are going to be evicted, or have their electricity cut off, or their benefit payments stopped.

In such cases, there may be appeal procedures that can be explained, or additional sources of help and advice that can be called upon. Such explanations can be hugely important.

Another area where explanations can be helpful is in interpreting and explaining other people's behaviour. Parents often become distressed with how their children are behaving; older people worry about the loss of various skills and faculties; members of minority groups may not always appreciate that the law is there to protect them against oppression and abuse. While there are no simple answers, sometimes an explanation, based on accurate knowledge and relevant research findings, can be very reassuring and supportive.

You should also not underestimate the importance of explaining what the law says, and what can be done legally to challenge certain decisions or actions. Some people, for example, value information about various pressure groups that exist to challenge aspects of social injustice, and welcome explanations about how they operate in the local and wider community.

Finally, it is becoming increasingly liberating to explain to people what information is available to them electronically, via the Internet and through various organisations' websites. The information explosion is both liberating and bewildering, and sometimes it is your role to explain to people which sources of information are most useful and, above all, reputable. It is, of course, dangerous to assume computer literacy, just as it is unwise to assume that everyone can read and write. So any explanations about the availability of electronic information needs to be tempered with a sensitive exploration about whether the person is able to access this information easily, or whether they would welcome being put in touch with a local organisation that can help them achieve this.

---

## Activity

Consider your own agency and the work you do. What are the key sources of information that are of most use and benefit to those who come to you? How do you make these available to people? What can you do to make these resources more accessible?

---

## ENCOURAGING

It is a truism to say that everyone needs encouragement, but in people-work it is particularly important to find and develop ways of encouraging people that do not come across as patronising, unrealistic or shallow. It is easy to overlook people's strengths and resilience when they come to see you and are overwhelmed by a particular set of difficulties. People-workers tend to get used to people who seem disempowered and unable to complete some mutually agreed tasks that were agreed at their previous meeting. It is tempting then to take over, and to begin to do things for people: it is often quicker, but in the long run it is counter-productive. Significantly, it risks undermining what self-confidence the person still has.

To encourage others, therefore, is a key communication skill in people-work, both among colleagues and with those who come to us for help. Try to find at least two things in each encounter or interview which merit a word of encouragement: this will be a huge motivation for future progress.

The words you use must be chosen with care. A glib, hearty 'well done' may be extremely patronising, and people will often know deep down whether or not they have given a particular task or undertaking their 'best shot'. Nevertheless, to say 'well done' at an appropriate point can be greatly appreciated, as can other forms of encouragement. For example:

'J, this is really good – I know you feel you struggle at times, but I think you've done really well doing this.'

'Not many people would have been able to do this, J.'

'I know you must feel disappointed at not having done as well as we had hoped, but well done for having a stab at it – it would have been easy to throw in the towel.'

'J, to have done this on top of everything else you have been worrying about is really good – you can feel proud of yourself.'

## ASKING

There are several ways in which sensitive questioning or asking can be an empowering experience. Sometimes this may involve stepping outside the immediate 'circle of distress' and asking some more general focused questions that can 'take the heat out of things' by trying to put the other person in touch with their strengths and resilience. It also helps you gain a fuller, better picture of the whole person, not just the presenting problems. For example:

- Ask people about what they are good at, and how they would normally handle a difficulty. This may produce a response that demonstrates their strengths but which also highlights the particularly disabling features of this problem that has temporarily got the better of them.
- Ask them in what way(s) they feel good about themselves, their life or their family, or what they enjoy most. This again may help them get back in touch with positive aspects of their lives that have temporarily been blotted out by their current problems. This has to be done sensitively: they may feel that there is nothing to report. You may need therefore to be gently persistent, but this is worth doing because it reinforces the value base of all people-work that you are seeking to communicate to them: that each individual is of value, worth and importance, and has inner gifts, strengths and the inner potential and capacity to cope, albeit with the help of other people from time to time.
- You can also gently ask questions about who has told the person in some way or other that they are not capable of dealing with difficulties. This is territory that can trespass into counselling and therapeutic interventions, which are not the domain of all people-work, so sensitivity is called for in exploring this theme. Nevertheless, in a low-key way, this question may be very revealing. People may begin to think back and reflect upon how their parents, or a teacher at school, or close friends, relatives or partners have 'put them down' and given them the message that they are 'no good'. This then provides you with an opportunity to challenge that perception, and to ask them whether they wish to continue to live under its domination, or to reassert themselves, to break out and take more control of their lives and actions. In some cases you may feel that a referral to a counsellor may be a very creative step for the person to take to 'kick-start' their personal journey towards liberation from these disempowering influences.

## TASK SHARING

There is a strong emphasis in people-work on the importance of partnership working and task sharing. This is for a very good reason. If you simply take over and do things *for* or even *to* the other person, however well meaning it may be, this risks undermining the capacity and confidence of the other person, and begins to inculcate a spirit of dependency upon you as the worker. Task sharing counteracts that risk by insisting from the outset that a pattern and a programme of shared tasks is negotiated by both of you.

The notion of a programme is important here. There are some situations where the person in need is so distressed and disempowered that you have to take responsibility for the first step of the journey. This may involve, for example, contacting the housing department over an eviction order, or a debt company to begin the process of review and repayment and putting everything 'on hold'. Similarly, someone with acute mental health difficulties who requires immediate hospital treatment will need the professionals to take responsibility to ensure that diagnosis and treatment are put into immediate effect. If there are overriding concerns about the protection and safeguarding of vulnerable children or adults, then steps must be taken without delay to ensure their safety. Someone seriously under the influence of alcohol or drugs may need to be kept safe until they return to a level of sobriety where they can begin to take serious responsibility for their future. The concept of a programme, therefore, is important because it includes the possibility of you having to act quickly and decisively, sometimes with the other person's consent, sometimes without it. At a later stage, however, the tasks will be more evenly shared and, towards the end, you will be the one who sits back because the other person will have gained sufficient self-confidence and resilience to take the lead and become more independent.

As the situation unfolds, therefore, you will want to begin to explore ways of sharing tasks in order to facilitate and empower the other person to take responsibility for their lives. The person whose lifestyle has become chaotic, resulting, for instance, in the non-payment of bills, will need to decide whether this is a downwards spiral from which they are desperate to escape. If that is so, then they will need to begin taking some responsibility for taking steps to achieve this, with your support. If they do not wish to escape, then there is little you can do apart from some immediate 'fire-fighting', because the situation will keep on recurring. People whose behaviour puts others at risk will need to begin to take responsibility for the consequences of their actions, and to decide whether or not they wish to change this cycle of disruption. If they do, then you can begin exploring parenting classes, offending behaviour sessions or anger management courses in which the person concerned begins to re-take control of their life to develop a more creative lifestyle which does not damage others. The person under the influence of drugs or alcohol similarly needs to make decisions about who or what is in control of their lives. It is not a decision that anyone else can make for them, but there are people like you who can share their journey and provide support and encouragement and skilled interventions.

The skill with task sharing comes in the negotiation and staging of the tasks that are to be mutually agreed. Too much too soon can be daunting and disabling; too little can be demeaning and off-putting. It is always important, therefore, to check with the person how they feel about the tasks that are being negotiated, and their capacity to deal with them. And when they report back, it is crucial to praise what has been accomplished, even if it is somewhat less than had been hoped for, and not to let setbacks be anything other than temporary. In fact, setbacks can be very enlightening because they throw up issues which perhaps had not been fully thought through beforehand when the tasks were being negotiated. An exploration into exactly why this task could not be fully completed may be very revealing for everyone concerned.

Implicit in all of this is the commitment you need to make to task sharing and partnership working. You need to be clear what you will be doing to help move things forward, and to ensure that you 'deliver the goods' by doing what you say you will do. But do also ensure that this process does not become competitive or point-scoring: it is all part of a restorative process to enable the other person to manage perfectly well without you.

## Group exercise

With the help of your tutor or supervisor, think about some of the people with whom you have been, or still are, working. Where on the spectrum of independency/dependency do you think they are located? In what ways have you negotiated task sharing? How far have you a clear picture of the programme you need to implement in order for the other person to become fully empowered and able to take full responsibility for their future?

## PROFESSIONAL RESILIENCE

At this point, we need to ask a fundamental question: how resilient are you professionally? It is all very well giving advice and guidance on how to treat others respectfully and in an empowering way, but in order to be an effective practitioner you need both to cultivate and maintain professional resilience. Otherwise you run the risk of burnout and losing that essential human spark that is at the heart of all people-work. All this talk about our capacity to facilitate others is based on the assumption that, as a worker, you are flexible, well-supported and sufficiently in tune with yourself that you are able to respond to others in creative and effective ways. Pressures of work, however, linked with personal difficulties that can beset all of us from time to time, mean that there will be occasions where your own resilience is undermined and your work with others impaired. Warning signs of these developments must be taken seriously. You need to take care of yourself if you are ever to be of any use to others.

There are several issues to consider here. First, do make sure that you take all your annual leave. This is part of your agency's commitment to you to help you remain fresh and responsive as a worker. The same is true for taking a lunch break. The pressures you face in your job will often make you feel that this is impossible, but unless you do take regular breaks there is every chance that you will begin to lose focus and momentum. Second, cultivate a professional support system. This could mean having one or two trusted friends at work on whom you can confidentially offload your worries and stress levels. It also involves a creative use of supervision, which is meant to be a vehicle for exploring areas of difficulty, as well as overseeing your caseload. You owe it to yourself, your agency and to those you seek to help to ensure that supervision meets your needs. Of course, there are some managers and supervisors in whom it is difficult, if not impossible, to confide on such personal matters, even when they impinge directly on your professional practice. Some colleagues fear that an admission of stress, for example, will be seen as a sign of weakness and an inability to do the job. In such situations, you need to seek out someone else in the organisation in whom you can trust so that you do not carry this burden alone. Finally, these themes need to feature regularly in how you and your organisation tackle your continuing professional development (CPD) and whether there are regular organisational health checks. Organisational culture plays a huge role in the wellbeing of workers and their capacity to work effectively. Indeed, an oppressive or bullying management style can quickly undermine the personal resilience of even the most committed individual worker.

## Work–life balance

Each of you will have your own strategy of self-care in your work–life balance. Taking time out, 'letting your hair down', having treats, enjoying sport and/or music, being pampered, enjoying intimacy: these are but some of the ways in which your batteries can be recharged. It is easy sometimes to feel guilty about having a good time when so many people for whom you are caring professionally are struggling. But, in the end, your effectiveness as a worker depends to a considerable degree on your resilience. Cultivate that, and your service users and patients will receive a better service from you.

## Activity

Develop a personal and organisational resilience audit. Make two lists under each of the following headings: SELF and WORK. Under each heading, list the positive activities and attitudes that foster your resilience. Then note the negative activities and attitudes that undermine your resilience.

You will want to be thankful for all the positives, but how will you deal with the negatives? Draw up an action plan to deal with one or two of the issues you have identified under each heading, with a timeline for what you hope to achieve.

# FINAL THOUGHTS

This section has dealt with important themes that lie at the heart of good communication skills – or rather, good communication skills lie at the heart of these important themes. It is all too easy to convey subtle messages of disapproval, and to invite a comparison between your success and the other person's failure to deal with life effectively. The communication skills necessary to foster the spirit of empowerment, and to tap into a person's resilience, are a mixture of the 'soft' skills of your attitude towards others and the value base you seek to embody, and the focused skills of active listening, interviewing and intervention techniques that can help you achieve your mutually agreed objectives. Everyone needs encouragement, and there can be few more rewarding situations than seeing someone regain confidence, resilience and the capacity to lead a creative, independent and fulfilled life.

## REFERENCES AND FURTHER READING

Carnwell, R. and Buchanan, J. (2008) *Effective Practice in Health and Social Care: A Partnership Approach*, 2nd edition. Maidenhead: Open University Press.

Department for Children, Schools and Families (DCSF) (2010) *Working Together to Safeguard Children: A Guide to Interagency Working to Safeguard and Promote the Welfare of Children*. Nottingham: DCSF Publications.

Greer, J. (2016) *Resilience and Personal Effectiveness for Social Workers*. London: Sage.

Saleebey, D. (2008) *The Strengths Perspective in Social Work Practice*, 5th edition. London: Pearson Education.

Thompson, N. (2007) *Power and Empowerment*. Lyme Regis: Russell House.

Thompson, N. and Cox, G.R. (2020) *Promoting Resilience: Responding to Adversity, Vulnerability and Loss*. New York and Abingdon: Routledge.

Trevithick, P. (2012) *Social Work Skills: A Practice Handbook*, 3rd edition. Maidenhead: Open University Press.

**RELATED CONCEPTS** acceptance; active listening; anti-discriminatory practice; confidentiality; counselling; emotional intelligence (EI); feedback (giving and receiving); non-verbal communication; spirituality; supervision

**ENGAGING WITH THE PCF** critical reflection; professional leadership; professionalism; values and ethics

**ENGAGING WITH THE NMC CODE** prioritise people; promote professionalism and trust

Service user snippet

Jolyon (54), unemployed, former drug abuser:

'I had given up – no job – no prospects – on the scrap heap I reckon … until Rick, my advice worker, took me in hand – for the first time someone actually believed in me, and what a difference that made. I began to believe in myself again and I've never looked back since.'

# ENDINGS

Best practice in people-work means keeping the ending of the professional relationship clearly in mind from the outset. This ensures that clear objectives are set, and that progress towards achieving them is clearly monitored and evaluated. It also ensures that once you have achieved your objectives, you will be able to disengage, acknowledge what has been achieved and say goodbye.

Endings are also important to consider with each and every meeting or interview you hold with the other person, so that the allotted time is used effectively. There is nothing worse than a worker giving implicit or explicit permission to someone to go into 'deep water', which may result in the person getting very upset as they try to make sense of painful experiences, only to be informed a few moments later that 'time is up' and they have to leave. There is then no time for them to regain their composure and return to their everyday world.

In both aspects of endings, there are essential communication skills: if they are practised well, the endings can be positive; if they are handled badly, endings can be upsetting and negative experiences.

## Activity

Think about some of the endings you have experienced in your life – they may be large-scale events or relatively minor. What impact did they have upon you? What do you think makes the difference between a good ending and a poor ending?

This Activity focused upon your experience of endings, not least because in people-work our own experiences often colour our approach to practice. How often have we heard people say that they do not like 'goodbyes'? Some will do anything to avoid those moments of 'closure'. For whatever reason, they are too painful, and perhaps stimulate within them some personal painful experiences of endings that they do not want to revisit. In saying this, we are not trying to pathologise some people's reluctance to engage with endings, but we are suggesting that, in this area, our own experiences may be a factor in how we deal with other, including professional, endings.

For some people it is the large-scale events that have cast their shadow. Experiences of tragedy and bereavement, for example, are losses on a grand scale that can seriously influence other less traumatic goodbyes. Like a spilled bottle of ink, their impact seeps into all sorts of hidden corners, so that even faint reminders of the pain are enough to make them 'fight shy' of other types of farewell.

This reinforces the importance of becoming a reflective practitioner. The situations you find difficult to handle, what scares you or makes you feel insecure: these aspects of your personality are not magically left outside the door of the interview room. They enter with you, and the secret of good reflective and self-aware practice is not to pretend that they do not exist, but rather to face them and to ensure that they do not encroach upon your professional dealings with others. This means that you have an obligation to yourself, as well as to those whom you seek to help, to explore these issues within supervision so that you can assess their impact upon your practice.

Again, for some people, this whole area of endings and goodbyes raises issues of 'existential angst', which is a rather grandiose, almost pompous, way of talking about what sense of meaning and purpose people find in their lives. Thompson captures this well when he talks of

> the type of challenges we face simply by being humans, by being in the world and seeking to make sense of it. Existential challenges can generally be seen as crises or turning points in our lives. (2012: 8)

These issues of meaning and purpose in our lives are part of the contemporary debate about spirituality, and form the backdrop to this issue of endings. This is not to suggest that as people-workers you find yourselves wracked with angst at each and every ending you have to deal with. That would be farcical and demeaning to your professional competence. But it does suggest that, from time to time, certain types of ending will 'get to you', and that this will often tell you more about yourself than the person with whom you are working.

This discussion takes us back to the importance of non-verbal communication; it is very easy to convey a set of negative messages about endings by your attitude towards them. But it is important that you make every effort to ensure that endings are positive for the people with whom you work, as well as for you as a worker. Some useful guidelines for achieving this include:

- Be clear from the outset why you are meeting together, what you need to achieve and how long this is likely to take.
- Keep your progress regularly under review so that you know how well you are doing and how near you are to completing your tasks.
- Be keen to offer praise to the other person for the progress they are making to help foster their resilience and independence.
- Do not be discouraged by setbacks – few people get it right first time, and there are things to learn from setbacks to help reach the ultimate destination.
- Remind yourself and the other person how much time you have left – this applies both to an individual interview (such as 'We only have 15 minutes left today – what do you think we can most usefully do in that time?'), and to the period of time set aside to achieve certain tasks (e.g. 'We agreed we would meet six times; today we are on session 4 – shall we review where we have reached and decide how best to use the remaining two sessions?').
- Allow some time at the end of each interview for the other person to regain their equilibrium if they have been upset. Try to normalise their re-entry back into their everyday life by asking a couple of ordinary questions about what they are doing for the rest of the day or week, and check that they are feeling all right.

- At the end, spend time acknowledging the achievements and progress made; affirm the other person's growing independence and capacity to cope; spend some time identifying how the person will cope in the future, and what other tasks may need to be dealt with some way or another.
- End the final session by wishing them well, and saying goodbye properly.
- Finally, write up your records, noting what has been achieved and how the 'case' has been concluded, so that anyone needing to find out about it in future will have a good accurate record.

## Group exercise

With the help of your tutor or supervisor, identify some scenarios where endings have been difficult for you. Using the guidelines above, discuss together how they might have helped you deal with the endings more effectively.

## FINAL THOUGHTS

It is often said that 'everyone likes a happy ending', but in your work with people that sounds a somewhat utopian aspiration. Nevertheless, your work should always have a purpose that is clearly defined and time limited, and if you make sure that you achieve at least a satisfactory ending to it, it will give a clear message that it is time for everyone involved to move on.

## REFERENCES AND FURTHER READING

Koprowska, J. (2014) *Communication and Interpersonal Skills in Social Work*, 4th edition. Exeter: Learning Matters.
Thompson, N. (2011) *Effective Communication*, 2nd edition. Basingstoke: Palgrave Macmillan.
Thompson, N. (2012) *The People Solutions Sourcebook*, 2nd edition. Basingstoke: Palgrave Macmillan.
Trevithick, P. (2012) *Social Work Skills: A Practice Handbook*, 3rd edition. Maidenhead: Open University Press.

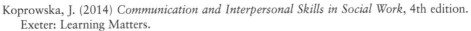

**RELATED CONCEPTS** empathy (dealing with upset service users); establishing a professional relationship; loss; non-verbal communication; reflective practice; spirituality

**ENGAGING WITH THE PCF** critical reflection; skills and interventions; professionalism

**ENGAGING WITH THE NMC CODE** practise effectively; promote professionalism and trust

Service user snippet

Marigold (37), user of mental health services:

'I was really getting on well with Gina my worker ... and was able to trust her I think, more than the previous lot ... and then suddenly she "upped and offed" without so much as a "by your leave". I was devastated.'

# ESTABLISHING A PROFESSIONAL RELATIONSHIP

It is often said that in people-work of various kinds, all that we really have to offer to someone else is ourselves. Our toolkit, if you like, is how we relate to the person who comes to us; in short, our communication skills. Whereas a car mechanic would be lost without a box of spanners and an electronic diagnostic machine, and a dentist without the range of drills, 'prodders' and fillings, people-workers are only effective when they have developed the skills to work with the other person in a professional human way.

Establishing a professional relationship is very much a communication skill in its own right, and includes a range of non-verbal communication skills. Perhaps one way of helping to clarify what is meant here is by stating what a professional relationship is *not*.

---

## Activity

Spend some time jotting down what you think should *not* be part of a professional relationship. Keep these notes beside you as you work through this topic.

---

As a professional people-worker, you are *not*:

- *A friend to the other person*: you will seek to be friendly towards them, but a friend often offers a far more comprehensive relationship than you can.
- *Always and instantly available*: you have responsibilities to other service users, clients or patients, as well as to other aspects of your organisation's work. You may sometimes decide to 'drop everything' to respond to a particular crisis with someone, but normally you will work within a system of mutually agreed appointments.
- *Offering general 'chat' sessions*: there will always be a clear reason for meeting in the first place, a clear set of objectives to work towards and a clear understanding of when the relationship needs to end.

- *Offering an open-ended relationship*: your time with the person will be focused on agreed areas of work, and for an agreed length of time. In fact, in most cases, the end of the relationship will be in sight at the beginning.
- *Offering a physical relationship to the other person*: we are much more aware these days of the difficult and at times compromising risks of physical contact between people-workers and those whom they are seeking to help. Physical contact can be misunderstood; people can be exploited when a sexual relationship develops between the worker and the other person. However mutually acceptable this may seem at the time, in fact it always constitutes a breach of the boundary of the professional relationship and therefore is always wrong.

This review of what is *not* a professional relationship is a helpful mirror-image to clarify what you do need to be aiming for when developing this with another person.

The most important aspects of establishing a professional relationship, therefore, are as follows:

- Always be clear yourself and with the other person about why you are meeting and what you need to achieve.
- Always establish clear boundaries, so that each of you knows what is and is not acceptable.
- Always be clear that you are representing your agency, and that you are accountable to your manager for the work you do; explain that this may sometimes involve another colleague sharing the work with you, or doing something on your behalf, or working with the person instead of you.
- Always be clear that the reward you will receive for your work will be in terms of satisfaction of a job well done. Receiving gifts from grateful service users should normally be tactfully declined – offers of money must always be refused. Sometimes, however, you may feel that to refuse a modest gift of appreciation, such as a bunch of flowers or a small box of chocolates, would cause unnecessary hurt. This is a matter of professional judgement, of course, but if you do decide to accept, say that you will take the gift back to your office for other colleagues to enjoy too. On your return, make a written note on the file and copy it to your manager explaining what has been given to you, and that this has been left at the office for general, rather than your own personal, enjoyment. Do check with your manager, however, about the team or agency policy on such matters, as this can avoid embarrassment or more serious repercussions (such as allegations of accepting bribes).

## THE PROBLEM OF TRANSFERENCE

You will also need to be aware of at least some psychological aspects of professional relationships. Whereas it is true that a judicious use of yourself can prove to be highly supportive, encouraging and even therapeutic for those with whom you work, there is a darker side of which you need to be aware.

When you become involved professionally with someone else, you never know what memories may be stirred up in the other person – or, for that matter, within yourself. How many times have we said, in our everyday transactions, 'Oh, you remind me of so and so', or 'You are just like …', or 'You sound just like …'. For all our uniqueness as individuals, we share some common traits and characteristics, and we all, from time to time, see other people in the face, voice, body language or behaviour of the person in front of us.

Most of the time, we deal with this without any difficulty – we see the 'connection' but then dismiss it, and refuse to let it cloud our dealings with the other person. But this is not always so. The psychological phenomenon called 'transference' is familiar to counsellors and psychoanalysts who work in-depth with people, and who sometimes find that their clients transfer onto them a range of deep-seated feelings, anxieties and needs. These can span a range of emotions from love to hate, and the worker has to be skilled at recognising when this is happening.

Within the more general spheres of people-work, such in-depth work is not part of your role, but nevertheless some degree of transference can still take place. As a worker, you may trigger some reaction within the person you are professionally involved with, not because of who you are, how you behave, what you say or how you look, but because something about you stimulates a memory within the other person, and they begin to respond to you *as if you were* that other person. Or they may begin to hope that you will be able to meet a deeper set of needs than is appropriate to your professional relationship.

Part of your professional response, therefore, will be to recognise that it is not *you as you* that the person is getting very angry about – it is someone else in their past who has caused them hurt which has not been resolved. It is not you they are falling in love with, but someone, or even some imaginary, fantasy person whom they hope will meet their deepest unmet needs. It is not you who makes them react to you as if you were an authoritarian parent; it is some parental figure in the past whose influence is still strongly at work at some deep level in their lives.

When we say, however, that it is not you doing this to them, that is only partially true. There is, of course, something about you that triggers this reaction in them, and you need to be reflecting and asking yourself what this might be. But you need to remain outside this reaction, and not to get drawn into it personally. If you are wise and perceptive, you will be able to work with these feelings and reactions to help the other person begin to understand them, and deal with them more effectively. You will realise that, in these situations, you are being given an insight into some aspects of what makes the other person 'tick', and this may help you tease out gently whether this sort of reaction to other people is common. If they can begin to see that transference is taking place, it may help them form more effective relationships in future.

There is another dimension. When someone you are working with triggers some unexpected and powerful feelings *within you*, you may find yourself projecting onto the other person something deep-seated within yourself. This is where self-awareness is crucial, linked to a supportive, perceptive supervisory relationship where such issues can be sensitively explored. This will help you to be set free to become a more effective worker. Often it is enough to realise, and to record, that some level of transference is taking place. To see it is to be able to stop it; it does not imply that you need in-depth counselling or psychoanalysis to sort it out. Just occasionally, however, the deep waters of your innermost self may be stirred and disturbed by such encounters, and you may then need to seek professional help.

Recording and supervision are important tools in helping you to recognise and deal with transference, both when it occurs in the other person and when it occurs within you. You may feel that a particular interview 'got stuck' for some reason, or that the other person's behaviour or reaction to you was a bit 'skewed' or odd, or strangely negative and resistant, and you wondered what was going on. Sometimes it is only in the post-interview reflection and recording that you can begin to work out what was happening, and how you can best handle it in future.

## Group exercise

With the help of your tutor or supervisor, think about someone with whom you have developed a professional relationship. Were there occasions within that relationship where you wondered 'what was going on'? Do you feel that transference was taking place in some ways? How did you handle it? How might you have handled it better?

## OTHER ASPECTS

There are further aspects to developing a professional relationship beyond the work you do with people who come to you and your agency. Two aspects will demand your attention: your professional relationship with your colleagues within your agency, and also with colleagues in other agencies. Each of these deserves careful attention.

### Professional relationships with colleagues within your agency

There are almost as many styles of team work among professional people-workers as there are people to populate them. If you have had experience of working in several teams, you will know that each of them has had its own unique culture. This will affect how colleagues relate to each other and to their manager(s), how they treat administrative and secretarial colleagues, and the extent to which team work is a stated objective to be worked at in specific ways, as opposed to a loose description of a group of workers who happen to inhabit a particular building. Individual characteristics quickly emerge in a team, and in larger teams subgroups sometimes form (referred to as 'cliques' by those who are not part of them); occasionally deep friendships are forged. Jealousies sometimes come to the surface, especially when there is a contested promotion opportunity; powerful personalities can seek to dominate other team members. By contrast, teams can also bring the best out of people by creating a supportive, creative and challenging environment in which individuals not only seek to do their best, but sometimes exceed their own expectations as the team culture strives for and achieves excellence.

Whatever your present team is like, there remains an underlying important principle to be observed: that you, and everyone else, must be committed to developing and maintaining professional relationships with everyone else in the team. This does not mean that you will necessarily like everyone or agree with them: that would be naive and unrealistic. But it does mean that you will need to do the following:

- Ensure that you know what your role is, why you are there and what your function is within the team and with those with whom your agency seeks to work.
- Avoid inappropriate relationships within the team: you need to treat everyone with dignity and respect.
- Avoid rumour-mongering, back-biting and 'putting other colleagues down'.
- Ensure that your own standard of work is always the best you can achieve.
- Ensure that other people can take over your work quickly and effectively if necessary: good, accurate and up-to-date record keeping is essential.
- Consult and seek advice where appropriate, and make effective use of supervision.
- Contribute to discussions and consultations within the team, making your own contributions clearly but respecting what others say, and ensuring that you carry out agreed decisions even if you do not wholeheartedly agree with them. It is not your job to undermine the team with niggardly negativism.
- Respect the agreed dress code and other cultural aspects of the team's behaviour. If you need to challenge aspects of this, do it in an open, honest way through team meetings or by raising it with your manager.
- Develop strategies for leaving your work worries 'at work' and not letting them distort your personal and private life.
- Give due regard to your own personal safety, especially when seeing people in their own homes or in unsupervised settings. If you work beyond the end of office hours and have not returned to work, make sure that you use the reporting system to inform your 'buddy' or designated colleague that you are safe and are going home. Make sure before you leave that the office staff know where you are going and what you are planning to do. This is for your own safety.
- Always plan for and take your annual leave entitlement. This is to ensure that you do not risk experiencing 'burn out', and that as far as can reasonably be expected, you are fresh and at your best to do your job effectively at all times.
- Notify your manager if there are issues of a personal nature that prevent you from doing your job properly. The boundary between 'personal' and 'professional' is not always easy to maintain, and if you are feeling particularly stressed or unable to function effectively, you owe it to yourself, your manager, your agency and to those who come to you for help, to be open and honest about this, and to see how you can best be supported through difficult times.
- Do not give out any information about any of your colleagues to anyone else, however plausible their request may seem. Personal information, including contact details, should remain confidential. You may offer to pass a message on

to your colleague, and ask the colleague to contact the enquirer direct. It may sometimes also be appropriate to give them a colleague's official work-issued mobile telephone number. But personal contact details must never be divulged. To do this would be a sure-fire way of losing the confidence and respect of your colleagues, who would have every right to lodge a complaint against you for unprofessional conduct.

- Note that there have been occasions in some teams where close working relationships between colleagues have developed into intimate friendships and sexual relationships. There are no absolute rules about this, but there are clear 'best practice' guidelines should this happen. These include: (1) notifying your manager about your relationship and being open and honest with them about it; (2) ensuring that personal and professional boundaries are scrupulously observed in the workplace, so that your relationships with other colleagues and those who use your agency's services are not compromised in any way.

## Group exercise

With the help of your tutor or supervisor, spend some time working through the checklist given above. This is especially important if you are a student about to go on placement or have recently joined a team. Draw up an audit of best practice. Discuss any glaring issues that cause you concern, and encourage other group members to contribute their ideas and suggestions.

### Professional relationships with colleagues at other agencies

This is a particularly important issue following the recent professionalisation of health and social care work, and the increased emphasis upon interprofessional working. The issue has come into even starker focus with the breakdown of trust and communication in tragic scandals such as the Mid Staffordshire NHS Trust, which resulted in the Francis Report (2013).

It is important to remember that each time you contact another agency in a professional capacity, you are acting as the 'face' and representative of your own agency. How you deal with others will, in some measure at least, confirm or diminish the reputation of your agency in the other person's eyes. Your professionalism (or lack of it) is therefore an important aspect of what you will be communicating to others.

How best to achieve this is not difficult, but it does involve following some basic guidelines. These include:

- State clearly who you are and which agency you represent. If meeting people face to face and for the first time, you need to present your ID card or badge to confirm your identity and show that you are bona fide.
- Observe all the professional courtesies about arriving at meetings/appointments on time, and observe the appropriate dress code.

- Ensure that you are well prepared: have key information at your fingertips, and say clearly why you need to be in touch with the other agency.
- Recognise and practise confidentiality. This may involve giving your contact details to the other agency for them to ring you back so that you can be verified as bona fide. After all, anyone can ring an agency and give false personal details and seek to gain confidential information. If in doubt, write a formal letter asking for the information you require on official letter-headed paper, or via a secure intranet.
- If you are leaving messages, give your name, your agency, the date, time and reason for calling, and remember to leave contact details for them to ring you back.
- Always do your best to return messages from other agencies as promptly as you can.
- If you have cause to complain about a colleague in another agency, seek advice and guidance from your manager beforehand so that you can be guided into the most appropriate course of action.
- Do not get embroiled in 'slagging off' colleagues from other agencies (or within your own agency), however justified you may feel because of their bad practice. If there are serious issues of malpractice, consult your manager in the first instance to decide on how most appropriately to act.
- If you are contacted by the press or media representatives about an issue, explain politely that you are not in a position to make a comment, but that you will ask a senior manager to get back to them if they give you their contact details.
- If you receive telephone calls asking for information about someone with whom your agency is working, remember the golden rule about confidentiality. Ask them to put their request in writing if you are unsure about whether they are bona fide. Always explain that you are not at liberty to divulge information about anyone without clear permission.

## FINAL THOUGHTS

The relationship you establish with someone whom you are seeking to help, support or advise in a professional capacity is crucial to the success of your work. If you get it right, then you stand a good chance of 'being part of the solution'; if you get it wrong, then almost certainly you will have become 'part of the problem'. It is as important as that.

## REFERENCES AND FURTHER READING

Day, J. (2013) *Interprofessional Working: An Essential Guide for Health and Social Care Professionals*, 2nd edition. Andover: Cengage Learning EMEA.
Francis, R. (2013) *Report of the Mid Staffordshire NHS Foundation Trust Public Inquiry.* Norwich: TSO.
Hammick, M., Freeth, D., Copperman, J. and Goodsman, D. (2009) *Being Interprofessional.* Cambridge: Polity Press.

Quinney, A. and Hafford-Letchfield, T. (2013) *Interprofessional Social Work: Effective Collaborative Approaches*, 2nd edition. Exeter: Learning Matters.

Thompson, N. (2011) *Effective Communication: A Guide for the People Profession*, 2nd edition. Basingstoke: Palgrave Macmillan.

Trevithick, P. (2012) *Social Work Skills: A Practice Handbook*, 3rd edition. Maidenhead: Open University Press.

Woodcock Ross, J. (2016) *Specialist Communication Skills for Social Workers: Developing Professional Capability*, 2nd edition. Basingstoke: Palgrave.

**RELATED CONCEPTS** confidentiality; emotional intelligence; endings; non-verbal communication; reflective practice; supervision; whistleblowing

**ENGAGING WITH THE PCF** contexts and organisations; professional leadership; professionalism

**ENGAGING WITH THE NMC CODE** promote professionalism and trust

### Service user snippet

Sarah (26), user of mental health services:

'I know this shouldn't happen but my worker reminded me of my first boyfriend and before I realised he made a pass at me and I let it happen ... I was feeling so lonely and needed someone to care.'

# FEEDBACK: GIVING AND RECEIVING

Feedback is the verbal or written evaluation of someone's performance; it is a comment on how well or otherwise they have done in completing a particular task. Effective feedback therefore requires excellent communication skills.

People-work provides many opportunities for feedback, as the following list demonstrates:

- A supervisor comments upon a trainee's interview which was formally observed and assessed.
- A senior nursing colleague comments on how you have dealt with a particular patient.
- A colleague asks you to say what you think of the draft report they have just written.
- Your manager evaluates your next six-monthly continuing professional development (CPD) plan, or your progress as a nurse towards re-registration.

These are but a few of the occasions where feedback is used, and almost always it carries with it the opportunity to suggest how performance can be enhanced or improved. In other words, it can be a valuable tool in promoting and facilitating best practice, assuming of course that it is given and received in the right way.

## Activity

Think about an occasion when you have been given feedback, perhaps as a student, or while developing a new skill or learning to play an instrument. How did that feedback make you feel? Was it constructive or destructive? What did you learn from this experience?

## KEY PRINCIPLES – ORAL FEEDBACK

How often have you been in a training event to practise some key skills when the person being asked for feedback on their own performance has immediately said 'It was dreadful' or 'I was hopeless'? The aspects of the interview that they feel did not go well immediately rise to the surface. But such nervous negativity rarely improves practice; it echoes the rather immature behaviour of a child seeking a parent's approval, comfort and reassurance, rather than an adult-to-adult, genuine quest for improvement.

The key principles for giving feedback, therefore, encourage you to take a different approach, both for giving feedback to someone else and also when evaluating your own performance. These principles are sometimes known as 'Pendleton's rules', and although developed originally in medical education, they are relevant to all people-work.

Pendleton's approach stresses that we can learn better if we first of all have the positive aspects of our performance identified and confirmed. Therefore, a typical first question to ask will be 'What went well in that interview?' or 'Tell me what pleased you most about how you conducted that interview' (Pendleton et al., 1984). This approach immediately invites you to think about positives, even if that feels a very difficult thing to do. There will always be things that went well, which will be strengths to build on. When these have been identified, then you can move on to ask not what was bad about it, but rather 'How might you have done it differently?' or 'If you had the chance to do this again, how do you think you might improve on what you have just done?'. This again puts the focus on best practice, and encourages you to think creatively about the skills you have used. Again, there will almost always be things which could have been done differently: after all, there is no such thing as a perfect interview.

The balance between these two approaches will vary. If, for example, someone has made a real 'hash' of an interview, or has given incorrect information, it would be foolish to spend too much time on the few positive aspects of it, leaving not enough time to focus on how the interview should be improved. People-workers spend their professional lives working with vulnerable people, and it is imperative that, particularly in the training scenario, maximum use is made of the opportunity to fine-tune these skills and approaches. Better that someone's pride is dented in the safe environment of a training event than making serious mistakes for real that could have been avoided had the trainer identified problem areas.

## FEEDBACK ON WRITTEN WORK

The same approach also applies to giving feedback on written work. It is always helpful to give an overall impression about the piece of work by saying what you particularly liked about the way it was written, its style or its clarity of thought. You can then move on to suggest how other aspects of it could be developed, or the style modified. Sometimes, for example, people forget the audience for which a report is being prepared. Formal reports call for formal language, whereas some letters need to adopt a far more conversational, informal tone to convey the right meaning.

Misspellings and poor grammar always need to be addressed. Usually, a light-hearted suggestion that they run this work through the computer's spellcheck or grammar check before sending it out will do the trick. But sometimes, when issues of dyslexia are involved, you need to check carefully that the person has had an appropriate assessment and has access to one of the many computerised packages designed to enable people for whom dyslexia is an issue to produce good, accurate pieces of written work.

## FOCUS ON THE BEHAVIOUR

When giving feedback you should always focus on the behaviour (e.g. the conduct of an interview) or the end product (e.g. a written piece of work), but not the person. Feedback is not an opportunity for character assassination; it is based on the assumption that the person will have done their best, albeit often in difficult circumstances, and what each of you wants from feedback is an acknowledgement of what went well and how performance could be improved.

Another important principle is that feedback should be given as soon as possible after it has been requested. If it is feedback on an interview, for example, the person giving feedback should try to give some immediate response as soon after the event as possible, using the principles outlined above. This could be quite brief, but it puts the person out of their suspense.

More detailed feedback can follow at an agreed day and time. If it is feedback on a written piece of work, there should be some discussion about when the feedback can be given and how. Would the person prefer this to be done verbally, or would comments written on the document be perfectly adequate?

## ROLE-PLAY FEEDBACK

The use of role play, especially with simulated patients/service users, is becoming increasingly popular in medical and social work education. This is because it is difficult for students in training to accurately play the role of a service user. It is far more authentic if an appropriately trained 'outsider' role-plays the scenarios. Feedback can then include a service user/patient perspective far more effectively.

Pendleton et al. (1984) suggest the following 'rules' or guidelines for such scenarios:

1   When the interview has finished, the interviewer is asked to comment on what went well, and this is followed by the role player giving their feedback, still in role. For example, 'As the service user/patient in this interview, I felt that you really made me feel at ease by the way you looked attentively at me, and asked me if I felt comfortable.'
2   Following this, the observer/trainer gives feedback, with specific examples of what went well.
3   The interviewer next has an opportunity to suggest what might have been done differently, and how certain aspects of the interview might have been handled in a different way.
4   This then enables the role player, still in role, to make their own suggestions for changes or improvements.
5   The observer/trainer can then add comments about how things might have been handled differently.

6    Finally, with the role player coming out of role, there can be a concluding discussion to clarify the learning points that have been identified. These points need to be specific and detailed so that the interviewer can use the feedback to improve on specific aspects of their performance.

These guidelines maximise the opportunity for constructive feedback, and can play a crucial role in helping trainees develop their communication skills.

---

### Group exercise

With the help of your tutor or supervisor, reflect on your previous experiences, perhaps while role-playing as part of your training, when you have been given feedback, or were asked to give feedback to a fellow student. How did this feel? What aspects did you like or dislike?

If you are a student you will often be formally observed by a trainer or more experienced member of staff whose role it is to help you develop your knowledge, skills and professional competence. Discuss with your group and your tutor or supervisor how feedback can best be given.

---

## FINAL THOUGHTS

This discussion is a reminder that you never work in a vacuum, and that communication skills are always a shared, corporate activity. We constantly need to check out whether what we are trying to communicate and achieve is actually working. Admittedly it is not easy to face criticism and to worry in case you have got it wrong. At such moments try to avoid a defensive default mode; instead, try to be open and honest about how you need to improve. The feedback mirror, therefore, is always an essential component in your 'toolbox', so that you can assess, with the help of others, how effective you are in the work you are undertaking.

## REFERENCES AND FURTHER READING

Pendleton, D., Schofield, T., Tate, P. and Havelock, P. (1984) *The Consultation: An Approach to Learning*. Oxford: Oxford University Press. See Chapter 5, 'Analysing interviews and giving feedback in experiential teaching sessions'.
Thompson, N. (2009) *Promoting Workplace Learning*. Bristol: Policy Press.
Trevithick, P. (2012) *Social Work Skills: A Practice Handbook*, 3rd edition. Maidenhead: Open University Press.

 Web resources

King, J. (1999) 'Giving feedback', *BMJ*, 318: S2–7200. Available at www.bmj.com/content/318/7200/S2-7200?variant=full-text (accessed 15/10/19)
MindTools (2016) 'Your top tips for giving and receiving feedback at work'. Available at www.mindtools.com/blog/tips-for-feedback-at-work/ (accessed 22/11/19)

**RELATED CONCEPTS** active listening; establishing a professional relationship; reflective practice; supervision; whistleblowing

**ENGAGING WITH THE PCF** critical reflection; skills and interventions; professionalism

**ENGAGING WITH THE NMC CODE** practise effectively; promote professionalism and trust

### Service user snippet

Jaswinder (20), nursing student:

'As part of my training I had to present a case summary to the team, and I was terrified. I thought I would have to wait until next week's supervision for feedback, and that worried me even more. But my supervisor took me to one side immediately after the meeting and reassured me that I had done well and that when we next met she would have some written comments to go with my own self-evaluation to help me learn from the experience. Whew, what a relief!'

# GENOGRAMS

The old saying that 'a picture is worth a thousand words' certainly applies to geno-grams, which are pictorial representations of a set of family relationships. With just a few basic symbols and a set of ground rules, you can quickly capture a lot of important information about the person or family you are working with.

Although genograms are usually associated with therapeutic family work, they can be useful for anyone working with people. They can be used both during and after an interview for the following purposes:

- To summarise the core information which has been gained.
- As a working tool to help gain information.
- To help understand and interpret information.
- To use in case notes to which other workers can refer.
- As part of an initial assessment interview with your service user, client or patient.

It is important to stress at the outset that anyone using a genogram during an inter-view must be very familiar with how it works, so that it really is a tool to be used and not a straightjacket which constrains. If it is not helpful to you, then don't use it.

## BUILDING BLOCK 1: LEARNING THE SYMBOLS

The symbols used in genograms are simple and straightforward.

Relationships are portrayed by lines that link the two (see sample genograms, Figures 4 and 5). A continuous line represents a stable, even permanent relationship, and a dotted line a recently established relationship that has not developed into any degree of permanency. If a relationship has ended, a single slash indicates a separa-tion; a double slash, a divorce.

At this point, some limitations will immediately become clear. There is no obvious distinction between a legally married couple and those who have been living together for a period of years. If it is important to know this, then you will need to add written information somewhere on or near the line (e.g. m 27/10/85 could be added for the date of marriage; cp 19/3/13 for the date when a civil partnership was legally recognised).

Already, two important points have emerged. First, pictures only tell us so much: we will need to add brief written notes to clarify or supplement information. Second, genograms can be used just as effectively for single-sex and heterosexual relationships.

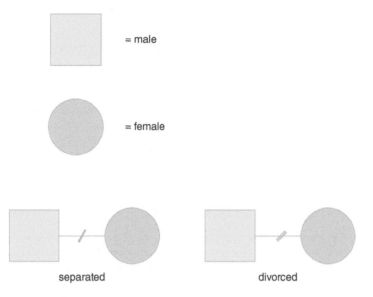

Figure 4　Building block 1

## BUILDING BLOCK 2: THE FAMILY TREE

Using the basic building blocks, a family tree can be depicted, with both children and grandparents being included. Additional information can be added to show the ages of the people concerned, and whether or not they are still alive.

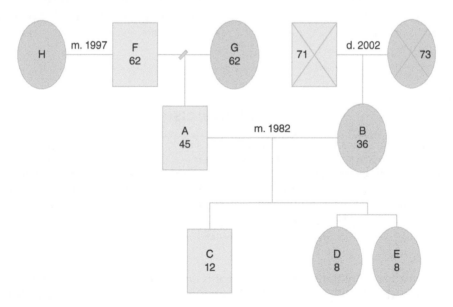

**Figure 5**　Building block 2

The genogram shown in Figure 5 tells us several key facts:

A is 45 years old, male and married to B, female, who is 36. They were married in 1982. They have three children: C who is a boy aged 12, and twin girls D + E who are 8.

A's parents F + G, both aged 62, are divorced; F married H in 1997, while G still lives alone.

B's parents are both dead; they died in 2002, aged 71 and 73 respectively.

---

## Activity

At this point, if you are not familiar with genograms, it is a good idea to 'have a go'. Start with yourself, and build it up in whatever way you wish, incorporating any siblings you may have; your parents and perhaps grandparents; your partner if you are in a relationship, and children if you have any. You will probably need a large sheet of paper to work on.

---

After you have completed your genogram, you should first of all check whether you have used the building blocks and ground rules accurately. This is important because, when you are using a genogram, another worker may *subsequently* need to look at it, and you will want to ensure that you are both speaking the same language with the pictures and symbols you are using.

The next thing likely to emerge is that it was probably not as easy as you thought. You may have wondered how to fit all the information in or you may have run out of space at the edge of the page and have had to start again. Don't worry, this is a learning curve and there is no rule to say you have to get it right the first time. So do make sure that you are familiar with how genograms work, and you will soon 'get the hang of it'.

## Group exercise

With the help of your tutor or supervisor, choose a Serious Case Review, or a report on a complex scenario familiar to your team, where there were several siblings and family members. Begin by analysing the information and family dynamics, and then with two or three group members begin to complete a genogram. Reflect on ways in which the genogram helps you gain a clearer picture of the family dynamics, and also how certain gaps in your knowledge may be highlighted.

One further thing to notice: sometimes it is only when we start drawing a picture that we notice the gaps and the details which appear to be missing – it is like an incomplete jigsaw, and it helps us to begin to ask questions about the information we have represented in our genogram. Who are, or might be, the people lurking in the background who still have to be mentioned?

You could, if this is an ongoing piece of work, take your genogram to the next interview or meeting, and explain that you have been trying to get a full picture of the situation. Explain how the genogram works, then ask them if this is an accurate portrayal; ask about the gaps which you think are there.

As soon as you start using a genogram *with* someone you are working with, tread very carefully. The information you portray in what may appear to you to be a very straightforward way in simple picture language, may have a powerful impact upon the person whose life is being 'examined'. The gaps may trigger off some emotional reaction when you start to explore them. So always remember that this is a tool that potentially can be very powerful.

The same point needs to be made if genograms are being introduced in a training context. You may find that the very process of seeking out information to complete the genogram can raise painful issues for some people.

## BUILDING BLOCK 3: INTERPRETING, MAKING SENSE, ADDING MEANING

The activities suggested above, and in the accompanying commentary, have taken us to the next level in the use of genograms: the interpretation of the information. This can happen in a variety of ways.

First, we may find that people want to talk with strong feelings about some of the characters who appear in the genogram. They may love them or loathe them, for example; they may feel very close to them, or very distant from them; there may be some very stressful relationships uncovered.

It is sometimes helpful, therefore, to capture these feelings and the quality of these relationships with some different symbols. For example, the use of a jagged *zig-zaggy* line between two people would indicate a very stressful relationship, whereas a thick, strong unbroken line between two people would indicate a strong – even affectionate – bond. And if you decided to use different colours on the genogram to emphasise these differing types of relationships, then a powerful picture quickly begins to emerge.

Second, some sensitive questioning about how various people in the overall picture relate to one another may again uncover some shades of meaning about the quality of the relationships and 'who means what to whom' in the overall family tree. By using the same symbols as before, an emotional, much more dynamic picture begins to emerge. Of particular significance may be the barriers between various people that block relationships. You may want to portray the barriers with a strong symbol on the genogram. If such barriers are problematic and trouble the person you are working with (and remember that the barriers may *not* be a problem, so it is not our job to make problems if they do not exist), then this may prompt a discussion about the barriers, how they feel about them and how they might be overcome.

Third, we can place a dotted line around all those who currently live together in the same household.

## FINAL THOUGHTS

It is implicit throughout all the discussion about genograms that you need to be clear in your mind about why you want to use them, and how they can be useful tools in your work with people. If you use them just for your own professional benefit, as an enrichment of your case recording, and as a means of reflecting on issues which have been, or still need to be raised, then you remain very much in charge of the process. Once you start using them in direct work with people, however, it becomes a much more interactive, dynamic, two-way process, where unexpected thoughts and difficult feelings may be stirred by this interactive process. That is its potential strength, but as a worker you need to be fully prepared emotionally for it to be a powerful tool in your professional relationships.

As with all tools, genograms have their strengths and their limitations. You may find that it will also be helpful to look at the possibility of using ecomaps, for example, when you are trying to explore more complex interrelationships between people.

The golden rule in all of this, however, is confidence. If you can introduce genograms into direct work with people in a sensitive, confident way, being aware of the potential benefits as well as possible pitfalls, then you are likely to find that the use of genograms can considerably enhance your practice.

## REFERENCES AND FURTHER READING

Coulshed, V. and Orme, J. (2012) *Social Work Practice*, 5th edition. Basingstoke: Palgrave Macmillan.

McGoldrick, M. (2016) *The Genogram Casebook: A Clinical Companion to Genograms: Assessment and Intervention*. New York: Norton.

McGoldrick, M., Gerson, R. and Petry, S. (2008) *Genograms: Assessment and Intervention*, 3rd edition. New York: Norton.

Web resources

LinkedIn Slideshare, 'Using genograms' – www.slideshare.net/JLSpicer/chapter-2-using-geno grams-to-understand-Family-Systems (accessed 15/10/19)

Multicultural Family Institute, 'Genogram life stories' – https://multiculturalfamily.org/publi cations/genogram-life-stories/ (accessed 15/10/19)

SmartDraw, drawing tool – www.smartdraw.com (accessed 15/10/19)

**RELATED CONCEPTS** ecomaps; empathy; reflective practice

**ENGAGING WITH THE PCF** critical reflection and analysis; skills and interventions

**ENGAGING WITH THE NMC CODE** practise effectively; promote professionalism and trust

## Service user snippet

Jason (12), living with foster parents:

'I like drawing and I liked drawing my family tree ... a genee thing ... and it was much easier to talk about mum and dad when I was drawing this picture with Jonny [my worker].'

# GETTING UNSTUCK

There is hardly a people-worker in existence who has not had the unnerving experience, while interviewing someone, of feeling completely and utterly 'stuck'. The interviewee has dried up and become silent, you have lost track of where the interview is going, you can't think of what to say next, and you wish that the ground would open up and swallow you. It is a very unnerving and uncomfortable experience.

Although there are no foolproof solutions, it is often possible to free the log-jam by using some tried-and-tested techniques before having recourse to the ultimate strategy of 'calling it a day' and deciding that no further progress can be made on this occasion.

Much will depend, of course, on the context of the interview. For example, an uncommunicative young person may feel overwhelmed by having to visit an austere office to meet someone old enough to be a parent or grandparent. In such circumstances, if no progress is being made, a change of venue or a younger worker may free up the communications. If, however, a person comes for an appointment under the influence of alcohol or other substances, it is wise not even to begin to interview them, but rather to give them another appointment and ask them to come in sober and clearheaded next time. There are also occasions when progress in an interview is minimal because the person you are seeking to interview is accompanied by someone who 'puts a dampener' on the occasion. A young person accompanied by a parent or relative may not wish to disclose information or feelings in front of that person and will retreat into a sullen silence to make precisely that point. In such circumstances, if alternative accommodation is available, and the setting is safe, the worker may suggest that just the two of them have some time together without the parental figure being in the same room. You may also find that on some home visits there are other people or children present, in front of whom the person you wish to interview quite appropriately feels unable to open up and discuss things with you.

These are some examples of where the experience of getting stuck – or sometimes of not even getting started – is due to circumstantial and contextual factors that need to be acknowledged and dealt with. Change the circumstances and you may well find that conversation begins to flow freely. Inevitably, this may mean abandoning the first meeting in favour of a second one in a more conducive setting, and this may annoy or frustrate you. But it is far better to recognise the barriers to communication at that point, rather than try to soldier on and find yourself becoming increasingly alienated from the other person.

There are also other 'barrier moments' that are more challenging, and will call for sensitive handling. For example:

- You are a white male worker and find yourself being asked to work with a married Asian woman.
- You are a black worker and find yourself in the presence of a white service user who 'point blank' refuses to be seen by someone who is black.
- You are trying to work with someone for whom English is not their first language, and who clearly struggles to communicate with you.
- A learning-disabled person with verbal communication difficulties becomes increasingly angry and frustrated at not being able to let you know what they need.

## Activity

Spend a few moments considering each of the scenarios outlined above. What do you feel is the best-practice response? Where do you think the barriers to communication lie in each of these scenarios? What strategies might be used to help them become 'unstuck'?

In these scenarios, it can be argued that in three of them the reasons for becoming stuck lie in the structural inequality of the relationship and the barriers that in some ways, wittingly or unwittingly, the worker erects. In such situations, best practice would suggest that an early attempt to remove such barriers will be a necessary precondition to meaningful communication. Ideally, a female Asian worker might be able to make significantly more progress than the original white male worker about whom the woman is likely to feel a strong measure of cultural diffidence and a reluctance to confide. With some Muslim women who choose to wear the burka, there are also issues of respect and cultural and religious sensitivity that you need to consider. Similarly, to provide effective communication assistance, by way of an interpreter or an appropriate communication board, may provide the breakthrough to better communication in two of the other scenarios.

More problematic is the situation where someone refuses a service on grounds of 'race'. Here the barrier is clearly located in the prejudice and racist attitudes of the person coming to the agency. The main question here is whether the agency should be seen to collude with these attitudes and provide a white worker instead, or whether the issue is so fundamental to the value base of the agency that they will say to the person that not only are such attitudes unacceptable to them, but also that the person must choose whether to accept the service from this worker or not to have any service at all. This is clearly an issue where the agency must have a very clear policy so that individual workers are fully supported in the decisions that are taken in such situations.

These are some of the contextual barriers that may cause you to feel 'stuck' when trying to conduct an interview. It goes without saying that until these barriers are removed to a greater or lesser extent, no meaningful communication will be possible.

Within an interview that has begun to make some progress, however, the possibility of getting 'stuck' is all too real. There are no automatic guaranteed 'unblocking' techniques, although some of the following 'tried and tested' approaches often yield some success. These are offered in no particular order of importance. The first two, summarising and paraphrasing, are basic skills you will want to use generally in your active listening skills, as they are useful techniques to facilitate progress during an interview, whether or not there are moments of getting stuck.

## SUMMARISING

It is useful when stuck to use the basic skill of summarising the story so far. You must find the form of words which suits you best, but something like this is what we have in mind: 'J, I wonder if it will help if I try to put into my words what you have been telling me?' and then after you have had an attempt at doing this, ask something like 'Have I got it right, J?' or 'Is that how it feels?' or 'Is this what you are trying to say to me?'.

The chances are that this will take some of the pressure off, and allow the other person to listen to you. In some ways, it does not matter if you do not get it completely right: they will quickly tell you if you have misinterpreted or misrepresented them, and that can give a fresh impetus to the interview.

## PARAPHRASING

This is a similar skill to summarising, except that with paraphrasing you do not need to try to deal with the whole story so far. Instead, you can take perhaps just the last point the other person was trying to make, and reflect it back to them in your own words. For example: 'J, have I got this right? You seem to be saying to me that you hate your father's guts?'

Again, this mirroring back provides an opportunity for the other person to discover how well you have been listening to them and how they have come across to you.

## ACKNOWLEDGING BEING STUCK

This may seem an obvious point to make, but sometimes it is the simplest things that work best. A range of statements or questions can be used to release the log-jam, such as:

'J, have you run out of things to say?'

'J, you seem really stuck – are you finding it difficult to continue? J, I wish I could help you carry on talking to me.'

'What is it, J? You seem lost for words.'

'Are you struggling with something really difficult to tell me, J? J, would you like a short break before we carry on?'

'J, would you prefer to carry on with this on another occasion?'

'J, I think you have done really well in getting this far – it doesn't surprise me that you want a bit of a breather.'

'J, is there anything else you want to say today?'

## SHARING THE SILENCE

Sometimes we fall into the trap of thinking that every moment must be filled with words. We find it hard to acknowledge that we find silences difficult to cope with, and that it is our needs which are being met when we want to kick-start the conversation as quickly as we can. It is just possible, however, that the other person's lapse into silence is no more, but certainly no less, than a pause for reflection. In such situations, you will probably help most if you stay quiet and allow the other person to have some space. Initially, no words are necessary, so long as you maintain a caring, interested body posture to help them appreciate that you are still 'with them' and are concerned for them. Judging when a silence probably needs to be broken, albeit gently, is a real skill, but you will gain some clues by the body language and general attitude of the other person. If they are clearly looking thoughtful and reflective and perhaps upset, it may be helpful to allow the silence to continue. You may also wish to encourage them with such comments as:

'It's OK to take some time out, you know. Take your time – there's no rush.'

'You've told me a lot today – perhaps it's important to be quiet for a while to see where we go next.'

'You don't have to talk, you know – it's OK to be quiet for a bit.'

'I'm glad you feel able to be silent with me – not everyone can do that.'

If, on the other hand, they are becoming restless, and are gazing round the room looking bored, that tells you that you need to re-engage quickly, and some of the summarising or paraphrasing techniques may help. But you may also want to face them with their apparent boredom in a direct way. For example:

'J, you are beginning to look a bit bored – have you had enough? J, can you help me – I'm not sure where we go from here?'

'Are you wishing you were somewhere else, J?'

'I suppose your teacher at school would've told you off if you'd looked as bored in class as you do now!'

'Come on, J – you're doing OK – let's have another go! Half time's over, J – time to come out for the second half! Are you still here, J?'

> ## Group exercise
>
> With the help of your tutor or supervisor, share examples in your group of occasions when you have got stuck. Using some of the suggestions and approaches in this chapter, try role-playing your scenario with another member of the group, and explore what approaches might help you to 'break the log-jam'.

## FINAL THOUGHTS

The very nature of people-work means that no one can tell you exactly how to deal with difficult moments like getting stuck; and perversely, no matter how much you seek to prepare yourself, when the moment comes, the feeling of being stuck is so real and genuine that it is not easy to break out of it. Nevertheless, it is useful to have some of these techniques up your sleeve so that you can 'oil the wheels' of the interview and help it come to a satisfactory conclusion. But if all else fails and you do not achieve a breakthrough, there is no harm in suggesting that you call a halt for today and arrange a further appointment. In such circumstances, it is helpful to acknowledge that you realise that they, and you, have found the interview difficult, and that next time you would like them to come prepared to talk about whatever topics or themes seem to be important. You might also like to pose a question for them to take away to help them prepare for next time. You can also offer to reflect on what might be most useful to think about next time, so that there is a sense of a shared responsibility for making next time become more productive for you both.

## REFERENCES AND FURTHER READING

Kadushin, A. (2013) *The Social Work Interview: A Guide for Human Service Professionals*, 5th edition. New York: Columbia University Press.
Thompson, N. (2009) *People Skills*, 3rd edition. Basingstoke: Palgrave Macmillan.
Trevithick, P. (2012) *Social Work Skills: A Practice Handbook*, 3rd edition. Maidenhead: Open University Press.

**RELATED CONCEPTS** active listening; barrier gestures; empathy; endings; interpreters; non-verbal communication; reflective practice

**ENGAGING WITH THE PCF** critical reflection; skills and interventions

**ENGAGING WITH THE NMC CODE** practise effectively; promote professionalism and trust

## Service user snippet

Andy (19), living in a hostel:

'I mean, we just sat there like … I dinna want to say much cos I was embarrassed so we just looked at the floor until my probation officer just stood up and said see you next week … what a waste of space.'

# GROUP WORK

'Group work' is a term that is used in a variety of ways which are not always clearly defined. At one end of the spectrum, there are therapeutic groups run by highly trained therapists who use the protected environment of a 'closed' group meeting to explore deep-seated issues for the group members, and encourage the participants to contribute actively to each other's therapeutic outcomes. Then there are various self-help groups where members share a common concern or problem, and support each other to overcome the difficulties they encounter. *Alcoholics Anonymous* is a good example of this. Within health and social care, groups are often used to bring together people who may need mutual support, or to tackle particular challenging problems such as anger management, spousal violence or changing offending behaviour. In such groups, the social worker or probation officer will take a lead in encouraging participants to tackle difficult issues in the hope that peer pressure and guided discussions will lead to behavioural change. Reminiscence groups for elders would be another example. At the far end of the spectrum, there can be an ad hoc gathering of a small or large number of people to discuss a particular issue or concern, where the energies and shared wisdom of the participants can be channelled into effective action.

## Activity

Make a list of various group work activities that you are aware of. What purpose do you think each of them fulfils? What sort of leadership and skills would be needed for the group to work effectively? How would you know if the group was being successful? Are there any dangers in such ways of working?

This Activity has encouraged you to begin to think more clearly about group work, what it is and what it seeks to achieve. You will probably have heard of Tuckman's (1965) 'stages' model of group work – *forming, storming, norming and performing* (he later added a fifth; *adjourning*) – which are useful to bear in mind not only as you think about preparing to undertake group work but also as useful concepts that provide insight into how groups often evolve and develop their own characteristics as they continue to meet.

If you think that a group-work approach could be a useful and effective way of working, the following key points are essential for you to consider:

1   Be clear in your mind about why group work might be a good way forward. Make a list of the objectives you hope to achieve.

2   Ask yourself who the group is for. Is it going to be for a specific number of people who will be invited to join for a particular purpose, or is it going to be open-ended for anyone to join? How will you advertise it?

3   How many sessions will be needed for the group to achieve its objectives, and how long will each session last? Who plans the content of the sessions?

4   What style of leadership is going to be needed to help the group succeed? Do you require an expert to give input and guidance throughout, or are more facilitative skills needed to enable everyone to make a valuable contribution?

5   What kind of venue will work best? How accessible does it need to be?

6   How will you know if the group has succeeded – or failed? How will you evaluate it?

7   What are the financial considerations? Does a venue need to be hired? Are travelling expenses or speaker's fees needing to be paid? Is membership of the group free or is there to be a charge? If so, is it the same cost for everyone or are some people to be exempt from payment?

8   Who will take charge of the administrative side of things? For example, publicity; agreeing dates; taking into account cultural and religious festivals that may impact upon attendance; booking rooms; taking enquiries; booking places; ordering refreshments and equipment; registering people on arrival; producing documentation; taking minutes or notes, if necessary?

These are some of the key points you will need to consider before any group work takes place. They can be summed up in one word: planning. Planning is an essential communication skill without which no group work could succeed. If you have ever attended a group session yourself where the leaders have seemed ill-prepared – no one is there to welcome you and to hand out information; the materials are not ready; the equipment has not been checked; and there is a general air of uncertainty or even mild panic – then you will know exactly why planning is important, and how disconcerting the lack of planning can be for the participants. It may only take a few moments to eat a slice of cake, but if the detailed preparation and cooking has not been meticulously undertaken for the appropriate length of time, then you will not enjoy the finished product!

The skills you will need once you have begun working with a group will vary to some extent depending upon the nature of the group. But in general terms, if you have a leadership responsibility for a group, you will need to focus on the following skills:

1   Be warm and welcoming in your approach to everyone involved to help them feel at ease and valued. Assume that people will feel nervous and anxious, especially in the first session, so think carefully about how best to put them at their ease.

2   Have everything you need ready to hand and be well-prepared. Check any equipment you will be using before the session begins.

3   Speak clearly and do not let your own anxieties make you gabble. Use clear plain English and check that you are being easily understood. Can everyone hear you easily? Are there some communication challenges you need to meet?

4    Keep to time, both at the beginning and at the end. People can get restless if events overrun, especially if they have transport concerns or family care responsibilities to meet.

5    Thank people for coming and find gentle ways of checking out that people are enjoying the group. An awareness of their body language and non-verbal communication can help with this.

6    Be prepared to rein in the over-eager talkative members, and to draw in those who find it difficult to participate in a group setting.

7    Be flexible. Sometimes a group needs to take a different direction from the one you had planned or expected. But also be prepared to bring them back on track if they get diverted and lose focus.

8    Be confident – or at least give the appearance of confidence even if inside you are feeling very shaky! People will respond to confident leadership. And if you can enjoy the occasion, so will they.

These are skills that are easy to list and far more difficult to put into practice. If you are not very experienced in group work, do try to link up with an experienced group leader to help you with your planning, and if possible observe them in action before you have to lead a group yourself. You will be surprised how much confidence you can gain by learning from others. And if you can share the leadership with someone else, so much the better, so long as you plan for this and know what each other is doing.

### Group exercise

With the help of your tutor or supervisor, work in small groups to plan a group activity of your choice (it can be hypothetical if you have not got a real scenario to plan). Begin with your aims and objectives, and plan everything in as much detail as you can. This will reinforce the importance of detailed planning, and will give you great confidence that a well-planned piece of work will be effective and enjoyable.

## FINAL THOUGHTS

Please remember that if group work is worth doing, it is only worth doing well; it could be counter-productive if it is done badly without the necessary planning and preparation. The more care that you give to getting it right, the more likely you will have a positive result.

## REFERENCES AND FURTHER READING

Doel, M. (2006) *Using Group Work*. London: Routledge.
Lindsay, T. and Orton, S. (2014) *Groupwork Practice in Social Work*, 3rd edition. Exeter: Learning Matters.

Preston-Shoot, M. (2007) *Effective Group Work*, 2nd edition. Basingstoke: Palgrave Macmillan.

Tuckman, B.W. (1965) 'Developmental sequence in small groups', *Psychological Bulletin*, 63 (6): 384–99.

Tuckman, B.W. and Jensen, M.A. (1977) 'Stages of small group development revisited', *Group and Organisational Studies*, 2 (4): 419–27.

**RELATED CONCEPTS** non-verbal communication; talks and presentations

**ENGAGING WITH THE PCF** contexts and organisations; diversity; professional leadership; skills and interventions

**ENGAGING WITH THE NMC CODE** prioritise people; promote professionalism and trust

## Service user snippet

Josie (23), living in a women's refuge:

'When we were told we were gonna meet as a group of women who had all experienced DV [domestic violence] I cringed – I didn't fancy telling my story to a group of strangers, like – no way! But actually it weren't too bad once we got going and I sort of realised I weren't alone any more … it sort of helped.'

# INFORMATION AND COMMUNICATION TECHNOLOGY (ICT) AND HEALTH INFORMATICS

People-work is about communication and the skills and expertise you require to achieve this effectively. Much of the emphasis in this book is on the human skills you need to fulfil your role, especially when working with people face to face. Whether it is dealing with someone facing a crisis, working jointly with a colleague or collaborating with other professionals, your communication skills are of paramount importance.

To do your work properly, however, you will need to be competent in a wide range of information and communication methods. Sophisticated developments with mobile phones, for example, make information and communication instantly accessible worldwide; social networking sites are now commonplace and an accepted means of social communication; powerful computerised systems store, process and analyse data swiftly and accurately. The organisations you work for will have developed their own e-systems for storing data and records, and some of them equip their workers with laptops so that records may be accessed and updated instantly. Within the NHS, GPs routinely check and update their patients' records on screen during the consultation, and developments in computerised technology allow patients to book appointments and choose a hospital of their choice for treatment. The use of text messaging to communicate with service users, clients or patients is becoming increasingly common. Without the skills to use these systems, therefore, you will not be able to do your job properly. ICT is now an organisational bedrock.

## Activity

To prepare for a future Group exercise, think about your own organisation. What contribution does ICT make? In what ways has it made your job easier? Are there ways in which it has made your job more difficult?

## Group exercise

With the help of your tutor or supervisor, find out more information about health informatics and information management (IM), and the contribution this makes, or could make, to your organisation. You may need to allocate certain tasks to each group member to research further information and then to report back to a subsequent meeting. Identify any future training needs in this area that you may have. Consider any recommendations to improve your agency's use of health informatics and IM you may wish to make in a report to your manager.

Against the complex and, at times perhaps, confusing array of ICT developments, health informatics has been developed as a discipline to help people make creative and effective use of the systems available to them, in order to help improve a range of healthcare problems. According to the NHS e-learning for health care, health informatics

> is the knowledge, skills and tools that enable information to be collected, managed, used and shared to support the delivery of healthcare and to promote health and wellbeing. (e-Learning for Healthcare)

At the practical day-to-day level of your work, there are some important guidelines that you need to follow if you are to use ICT effectively without falling into some of the traps that await the unwary. These include:

- As a professional people-worker, you need to be aware of the policy guidelines, rules and procedures about ICT in your organisation. There will be strict rules about confidentiality, for example, and what you may or may not do when using office equipment and systems. The ICT facilities provided by your agency are for the benefit of the agency, its employees and those whom it seeks to serve. It is not there as an extension to your private email or social website for you to use for your personal benefit or gain.
- Inappropriate use of emails (e.g. to harass others, cause offence, or if written in disrespectful language) is unacceptable, as is sending out or passing on offensive messages or materials. You should also be careful about circulating seemingly innocuous 'jokey' material from your work email address. This is not meant to sound mean-spirited or to deny the value of humour, but to encourage you to check with your organisation what its policy and guidelines are, and not to open yourself up to grounds for complaint.
- You need also to be careful about emails asking you for personal information, or warning about 'scams' currently in operation. Sometimes these release viruses if opened. When in doubt, do not open them or pass them on, but seek advice from your IT department.
- Check your organisation's house style and expectations about the use and format of emails. Good *netiquette* requires you to observe all appropriate protocols such as stating the subject of your email; ensuring that your personal signature

details are correct; being concise without being terse. Pay careful attention to the tone of your email; you could easily give the wrong impression by an inappropriate choice of words or how you phrase a request, or by sending a message in capital letters, which suggests that you are 'shouting'. Only copy people in who need to be included: to receive unnecessary copies of other people's emails can be frustrating and time-consuming.

- You will be using the Internet as part of your work, often to research and access important information. You should be aware, however, that to surf the Internet for pornographic material or to conduct online personal shopping could lead to disciplinary procedures.

- Seek permission before you bring your own memory stick or CD material into work. Some organisations are very strict about this in order to protect their systems against virus attack.

- Never use your home computer for confidential work purposes. This would be a clear breach of the Data Protection Act 2018 and could seriously jeopardise your code of confidentiality.

- Social websites are increasingly popular, and as an individual you may make regular use of them. The boundary between *personal* and *professional*, however, is not always watertight, and you need to think twice before putting certain pictures or information about yourself onto Facebook or YouTube, for example, which could cause you embarrassment or worse, if it became known to your employer.

- Many organisations now encourage their employees to use text messaging as part of their work practice, including contacting the people with whom they work, or to send out important information. This is quite common, for example, when working with young people. Similar protocols apply here as for the use of emails. It is important that you maintain your professional approach with all your communications, even if some of them need to be light-hearted.

- Official communications often still need to be in writing and sent to people in the post, even though this may feel time-consuming compared with email or texting. Your organisation will have a policy about this and you must check carefully so that you act appropriately. There are sometimes legal implications involved.

- You must be sure that the person with whom you are communicating can understand what you are saying, whether this is in writing, by email or texting. English may not be their first language, for example, and you may need an interpreter. People's reading skills vary, so you should find sensitive ways of checking that they understand what you have written. This is particularly important if you are asking them to read through and approve or modify a formal report you have prepared for court or a case conference, for example. It is your responsibility to check that they understand. On occasion, you may need to read the report out to them in a private setting two or three times to ensure they have grasped its full meaning and significance. People who have learning difficulties, or who are deaf or visually impaired, will need you to take particular care to ensure that you are communicating with them effectively and on their own terms.

- Finally – you all use jargon and acronyms as part of your daily work. They help you as professionals to communicate easily. But they can bewilder and perplex those who are outside your circle. Think twice; use plain English, and check that the other person really has understood what you are saying.

---

## Group exercise

With the help of your tutor or supervisor, in small groups work through the above checklist. Go through each item in turn and relate it to your own practice, both as an individual and within your organisation. Are there any topics you would wish to add to this list?

---

## FINAL THOUGHTS

Advances in information technology and health informatics have developed with breathtaking speed. They have already enriched our capacity to provide effective services and to deepen the knowledge and research base for our work. We have amazing tools at our command. But there are risks involved, and as a professional you must be in control, and not put yourself or your organisation at risk by inappropriate involvement with social media sites. We do inhabit a different country, but the ethics remain the same.

## REFERENCES AND FURTHER READING

Dickson, N. (2014) Cited in a conference presentation by Dr Ben Riley (RCGPs) on the *Social Media Highway Code*, Keele University Medical School, 23 March.

e-Learning for Healthcare 'About the Health Informatics programme'. Available at www.e-lfh.org.uk/programmes/health-informatics (accessed 22/11/19).

Englebardt, S. and Nelson, R. (2002) *Health Care Informatics*. St Louis, MO: Mosby.

Nelson, R. and Staggers, N. (2017) *Health Informatics*, 2nd edition. Amsterdam: Elsevier.

Rafferty, J. (2007) 'Social work in a digital society', in M. Lymbery and K. Postle (eds), *Social Work: A Companion to Learning*. London: Sage.

Riley, B. (2013) *The Social Media Highway Code*. London: Royal College of General Practitioners. Available at www.rcgp.org.uk/social-media (accessed 15/10/19).

Sullivan, F. and Wyatt, J.C. (2006) *ABC of Health Informatics*. London: Blackwell/BMJ.

Watling, S. and Rogers, J. (2012) *Social Work in a Digital Society*. Exeter: Learning Matters.

---

**RELATED CONCEPTS** interpreters; learning difficulties; telephone skills

**ENGAGING WITH THE PCF** contexts and organisations; professionalism; values and ethics

**ENGAGING WITH THE NMC CODE** promote professionalism and trust

## Service user snippet

Annabelle, nursing graduate:

'I was completely overwhelmed by information overload and how to make sense of it for my organisation. Fortunately a course on Health Informatics opened the door for me and at least I can find my way around now.'

# INTERPRETERS

In a multicultural society, there is an increasingly important emphasis to be placed on the availability of interpreters so that people for whom English is not their first language may have their needs and requirements accurately addressed.

Interpreting, of course, is a much wider communication than this initial definition suggests. In any communication between and among people, there will be a continual process of interpreting as we try to make sense of what the other person is seeking to communicate. How we interpret non-verbal communication or barrier gestures are good examples of this: we need to check whether the meaning we are applying to their message is accurate or not; or, to put it another way, whether we are accurately interpreting what the other person is saying or doing. Interpreting therefore is a fundamental, generalist skill that underlies and underpins all communication.

This skill comes into sharper focus, however, when issues around language are involved. Not only are there the general challenges of understanding what the other person is saying; there is also the added challenge of translating this message from one language to another in order for it to be properly received.

---

## Activity

Think about the work you do and the demographic make-up of the area your agency or hospital covers. Do you know how many different cultural groups there are, and therefore how many different languages are in general use in the area? Do you know how many people are not able to converse with agencies using English? How many would much prefer to have the use of a skilled interpreter so that they can explain what they need in their first language? If you find these questions difficult to answer, contact your local authority and obtain a copy of the latest census, which will reveal many of the answers.

---

Your responses to the above Activity will have been informative, and will have given you some idea of the size and scope of the challenge your agency faces. There is considerable political debate, of course, about the extent to which everyone in the UK should have a sufficiently clear grasp of English in order to access services effectively. But the issue is more complex than that. In Wales, for example, it has been a matter of pride and national/cultural identity that people should be given the choice as to whether they access information and services in Welsh or English. It is a similar principle and value base that is behind the drive to extend this choice to other cultural groups within society.

There are additional issues to consider. Deaf people, for example, for whom British Sign Language (BSL) is their first language, do not have the option of linguistic choice. BSL is their language, and there is a responsibility and legal obligation upon organisations to ensure that Deaf people can access information and services.

British Sign Language is a good example to explore because it highlights some of the key issues of interpretation, and indeed translation, that underlie all attempts to convey meaning accurately from one language to another. With BSL, there is a structural issue to take into account because it is such a visual means of communication. The most obvious example that is familiar to anyone learning basic BSL is how you ask someone else's name. 'What's your name?' seems an easy enough question to pose, but in BSL the literal translation would be 'Your name, what?' because the visual message needs to have a different structure in order to make it more quickly comprehensible. A system of 'multichannel' signs in BSL ensures that a broad range of complex communication can be shared quickly and easily without having recourse to a laborious fingerspelling of every single word.

For someone to be an effective interpreter for a Deaf person, therefore, they not only need a deep knowledge of two languages, but also an ability to move between them quickly and fluently so that the real meaning behind the words or symbols can be effectively communicated.

This example illustrates the complexity of an interpreter's task. In some languages and cultures, there may not be an equivalent or comparable word for such terms as 'depression', 'dementia' or 'counselling', for example, and the interpreter may have a difficult task in trying to convey and translate what is meant. Indeed, there may have to be a discussion between the worker and the interpreter so that the worker is 'brought up to speed' with the problems that certain words, terms and phrases are causing (Williams and Abeles, 2004).

This highlights two key principles behind all interpreting: trust and accuracy.

## TRUST

The issue of trust is paramount, and is two-sided. For example, a woman whose first language is Punjabi may be accompanied by her husband or another male family member who will act as interpreter for the interview. There is no doubt that if that family member has a command of English, good interpretation is possible. But a female worker may feel that issues of gender and culture may become a barrier to accurate communication. She may not be sure whether the male family member is putting across his own interpretation or opinion rather than accurately conveying what the woman is actually saying. She may begin to wonder whether she can really trust the process of interpretation.

For this reason, it is considered best practice in all people-work for an official, accredited interpreter to be made available for such interviews, and indeed for other official and formal occasions such as court appearances or meetings with local authority officials. The interpreter's code of conduct should ensure that good accurate communication takes place, especially as factors such as gender and 'race' are taken into account in the choice of interpreter to be employed for this purpose.

There can, of course, be no absolute guarantee of this, not least because communication is such a complex phenomenon. But every agency should have access to an interpreter scheme to ensure that these basic issues can be properly and effectively addressed, and that both 'parties' feel that they can trust the interpreter to do the job honestly, accurately and without any personal prejudice.

## ACCURACY

The principle of accuracy is also fundamental, and underlies the capacity of each person to understand the other. From the worker's point of view, it is important to establish some appropriate guidelines and ground rules before an interview or meeting begins. These include:

- checking that the other person is happy with the interpreter and can trust them to communicate their views and opinions honestly and accurately;
- checking that the interpreter knows the ground rules and code of conduct, and is willing to translate and interpret accurately, even if the views and opinions that are being interpreted go against their own personal or cultural convictions;
- agreeing the boundaries and whether it is acceptable for the interpreter to begin to plead the cause of the other person in addition to the role of the interpreter, and to be clear when this is being undertaken;
- explaining the structure of the interaction, by giving an undertaking that the interview will not be hurried, that the conversation will be conducted in easily manageable 'bite-size chunks', and that on a regular basis the worker will pause to check that everything is clear;
- encouraging the other person to say at any point if they do not understand what is being said or asked of them;
- encouraging written notes to be made in each language about key points being made; it is good practice for each person to have a copy of the notes in each language for future reference.

Working with interpreters is an important skill that needs practice. It is useful to discuss this with colleagues who have already developed these skills, and if possible to seek permission to sit in on and observe another interview where an interpreter is being used so that you can 'get the feel' of what is involved before you have to do it 'for real' yourself.

### Group exercise

With the help of your tutor or supervisor, can you discover the interpreting needs of the community your agency is serving? Do you have an up-to-date register of interpreters? If not, it will be an important project for your team to research and produce one.

## USER PERSPECTIVES

A criticism of the discussion so far could be that it seems to be from an agency or service provider perspective; it might even be argued somewhat cynically that these procedures are there to 'cover the backs' of the professional workers in case things go wrong. Such a response would be unwarranted and unfair: best practice is best practice, and there are good reasons underpinning the approaches that have been outlined so far. Nevertheless, any approach that does not fully take into account the user's perspective is bound to feel somewhat 'one-sided', and a negation of the basic principle of partnership working at the heart of all people-work.

Some important research was conducted by Alexander et al. (2004) with multi-cultural communities in London and Manchester. Their findings highlighted some important issues for all people-work by drawing attention to the following responses from people who needed interpreters:

- The decision about whether or not an interpreter was necessary should be decided by the people themselves, depending on the situation they were facing. Often they felt they could manage perfectly well by themselves or with their own chosen interpreter, but in legal and medical matters the importance of a trained interpreter was emphasised.
- People expected their interpreters to have good people skills, and where necessary to be able and willing to 'go the extra mile' and plead their cause for them. The personal qualities of trustworthiness and reliability were seen to be crucial. Where these qualities were clearly evident, high expectations were placed on the interpreter to be an effective advocate as well as an interpreter, and to achieve results from a service provider agency which they feared seemed better at with-holding services than granting them.
- There was considerable difficulty in accessing good-quality interpreters in these areas, so that many people preferred family and friends to undertake this role because they felt they could rely on their loyalty and emotional commitment.

These findings demonstrate how important it is for there to be an open and honest dialogue right at the outset to explore the issues of trust and accuracy, what is going to work best for the other person, and also what is best going to serve the legitimate needs of the agency. The worker needs to check carefully that the interpreter can communicate with and understand the person, and vice versa, and that they will faithfully do their job without putting their own interpretation on what is being said. Likewise a service user or patient may find it convenient sometimes to pretend not to have understood what was being said. It is important therefore that at an early stage the worker records accurately how the interaction between everyone involved is understood and practised. To use a professional interpreter when the worker and the person they are working with have different racial backgrounds is another key consideration when English isn't their first language. To explore these issues effectively will require good communication and listening skills, but if handled sensitively will ensure that a good outcome can be achieved.

## Group exercise

With the help of your tutor or supervisor, discuss what skills and strategies you will need to ensure that the service user's/patient's 'voice' is heard.

## FINAL THOUGHTS

Perhaps the only way in which you will fully understand the importance of inter-preters is to be in a situation where you need one yourself – perhaps on holiday in a country where you do not speak the language and have some sort of crisis. You will then need to have someone who is able to help you to become fully involved in the negotiations so that you know exactly what is happening and what is involved. That perhaps will give you an insight into how important good-quality interpreting is at both the emotional and the practical level.

## REFERENCES AND FURTHER READING

Alexander, C., Edwards, R. and Temple, B., with Kanani, K., Zhuang, L., Miah, M. and Sam, S. (2004) *Access to Services with Interpreters: User Views*. York: Joseph Rowntree Foundation.

Green, J., Free, C., Bhavnani, V. and Newman, T. (2005) 'Translators and mediators: Bilingual young people's accounts of their interpreting work in health care', *Social Science and Medicine*, 60 (9): 2097–110.

Herndon, E. and Joyce, L. (2004) 'Getting the most from language interpreters', *American Academy of Family Physicians Family Practice Management*, 11 (6): 37–9.

Koprowska, J. (2014) *Communication and Interpersonal Skills in Social Work*. London: Learning Matters/Sage.

Williams, C.R. and Abeles, N. (2004) 'Issues and complications of deaf culture in therapy', *Professional Psychology: Research and Practice*, 35 (6): 643–8.

Woodcock Ross, J. (2016) *Specialist Communication Skills for Social Workers: Developing Professional Capability*, 2nd edition. Basingstoke: Palgrave Macmillan.

Web resource

Kwintessential, Translation agency – www.kwintessential.co.uk (accessed 11/09/19)

**RELATED CONCEPTS** active listening; anti-discriminatory practice; empathy; establishing a professional relationship

**ENGAGING WITH THE PCF** contexts and organisations; professionalism; skills and interventions; values and ethics

**ENGAGING WITH THE NMC CODE** practise effectively

## Service user snippet

Mohammed (16):

'I didn't know what to say to all these people asking me where I had come from and how I had got into the UK. But thank god for the interpreter who put me at my ease and made sense of everything. I would have been lost without him.'

# INTERPROFESSIONAL COLLABORATION

Wherever your professional allegiance and expertise may lie, contemporary people-work will require you to work effectively and professionally with other colleagues and agencies. This requirement is partly driven by the truism that *two (or more) heads are better than one*. If other colleagues have experience, knowledge and expertise that can enrich your own contribution, or if you can add an important ingredient to the mix with other agencies, then it makes sense for this to happen so that the service user/client/patient who is at the receiving end can receive the best possible service. The next step, of course, is to ensure that within any partnership or collaborative working, the service user/client/patient is also fully involved in this process.

Your professional body will most likely have a policy statement about this issue that ensures that interprofessional collaboration is not just a good idea, but is enshrined in everyday practice.

---

## Activity

Discover what policy statements your organisation has made about interprofessional collaboration. Are there any boundaries or limitations to such collaboration from your agency's point of view?

---

To give you a flavour of such statements, Preston-Shoot (2009) notes that:

> The benchmark for medicine (Quality Assurance Agency, 2002) requires doctors to be able to work with other healthcare professionals, to give appropriate input to multidisciplinary teams and to promote effective interprofessional partnerships.

Contemporary social work practice increasingly takes place in an interagency context. Social workers must be skilled in consulting actively and acting collaboratively with others, negotiating across differences such as organisational and professional boundaries (Preston-Shoot, 2009: 32–3).

Another powerful driver towards interprofessional collaboration is to be found in the official reports arising out of the tragic deaths of children such as Victoria Climbié (Laming, 2003), and various Serious Case Reviews. Time and again, professional lack of collaboration has been highlighted as a major obstacle that needs to be overcome if adequate safeguarding and protection is to be achieved, not just for children but also for vulnerable adults.

## Group exercise

With the help of your tutor or supervisor, identify a Serious Case Review where issues of interprofessional collaboration have been highlighted. In small groups develop an ecomap with a focus on the various agencies, support systems and resources involved with this particular family. Identify what mistakes were made and any obstacles you think hindered interprofessional collaboration. What picture does your ecomap reveal about best practice and lessons to be learned?

In your group exercise, you will have begun to unravel some of the complexities of interprofessional collaboration. Some of these considerations will include:

- There can be real dilemmas about your obligation to maintain confidentiality and the extent to which information may be shared with other agencies. Data protection legislation and protocols have added to the complexities of information sharing.
- There can be a lack of awareness of which other agencies/colleagues may be involved and how they can contribute to an outcome.
- Sometimes agencies are divided by a common language; does everyone mean the same thing when they use words like 'prevention', 'intervention', 'protection', 'assessment', 'holistic practice'?
- Is there a meeting point between the medical and social models of care?
- Who pays for whom to do what?
- With whom does the buck ultimately stop?
- Professional training often *fails* to include interprofessional issues.
- How do we ensure that the service user/client/patient is allowed to be centre stage?
- Can we trust colleagues in the voluntary sector?
- It takes too much time to arrange all these meetings!

These considerations and many more you may have been able to identify are intended to be nothing more than a 'reality check' for your own practice, at whatever stage you are at in your professional development. It may sometimes feel like you are *between a rock and a hard place* with this issue of interprofessional collaboration. Certainly there are no easy answers, but here are some guidelines to help you:

- Never rush in – spend some time carefully thinking through in a reflective way about the best way forward. Even your responses to urgent crises need to be thought through carefully.

- Always be very clear about your own role, the role of your agency and to whom you are accountable.
- Always keep the service user/client/patient at the forefront of your thinking.
- Ask yourself who else needs to be involved, what expertise they could bring and what might happen if they were not involved.
- Start with interprofessional collaboration as your 'default position' and only veer away from that if there are compelling reasons to do so.
- Always talk matters through with your line manager/supervisor if you are uncertain about how best to proceed.

Please keep in mind a service user or patient perspective. Whenever a service user or patient attends a meeting with many professionals in attendance, please make sure they know who is there, what service or organisation they represent, and what their particular role is. They need also to be aware that although there may be differences of views and opinions between professionals, these should be aired professionally to ensure that the service user/patient maintains confidence in those who are working with and supporting them.

## FINAL THOUGHTS

As a worker you may sometimes feel that other professionals may be trying to undermine your approach, values or strategy, which can lead to feelings of frustration or may undermine your professional confidence. Try not to take this personally or become defensive or aggressive; always explore what is in the service user's or patient's best interest, and take any difficult feelings you may have back to supervision. It is also worthwhile giving serious consideration to opening up conversations with other professionals who you may feel are undervaluing your professional contribution and role. There may be a genuine misunderstanding; but in any case open, honest discussions, based on a shared understanding of what is in the service user's or patient's best interests, will help to build solid foundations for your continuing interprofessional working relationships.

If ever you feel that this aspect of your work is too time-consuming, remember the increasing number of official reports into various tragedies which point to the lack of interprofessional collaboration as a major factor in the failure to prevent the tragedy from happening. People's lives are at risk.

## REFERENCES AND FURTHER READING

Barrett, G., Sellman, D. and Thomas, J. (2005) *Interprofessional Working in Health and Social Care: Professional Perspectives*. London: Palgrave Macmillan.
Hammick, M., Freeth, D., Copperman, J. and Goodsman, D. (2009) *Being Interprofessional*. Cambridge: Polity Press.
Laming, Lord (2003) *The Victoria Climbié Inquiry*. Norwich: HMSO.

Preston-Shoot, M. (2009) 'Repeated history? Observations on the development of law and policy for integrated practice', in J. McKimm and K. Phillips (eds), *Leadership and Management in Integrated Services*. Exeter: Learning Matters.

Quality Assurance Agency (2002) *Medicine*. Available at www.qaa.ac.uk/Medicine (accessed 20/03/17).

Quinney, A. and Hafford-Letchfield, T. (2012) *Interprofessional Social Work: Effective Collaborative Approaches*, 2nd edition. Exeter: Learning Matters.

Trevithick, P. (2012) *Social Work Skills and Knowledge: A Practice Handbook*, 3rd edition. Maidenhead: Open University Press.

Wallace, C. and Davies, M. (2009) *Sharing Assessment in Health and Social Care: A Practical Handbook for Interprofessional Working*. London: Sage.

**RELATED CONCEPTS** chairing meetings; ecomaps; establishing a professional relationship; values and ethics

**ENGAGING WITH THE PCF** context and organisations; critical reflection and analysis; professionalism

**ENGAGING WITH THE NMC CODE** practise effectively; promote professionalism and trust

## Service user snippets

Leroy and Maddie (both 22), parents:

'We had to attend this meeting about the kids and the room was full so we were dead scared. But Leo, our worker, explained who everyone was and that they were all there to help us with the kids … we didn't realise they all worked together like that, and it all got sorted. Great!'

Gabriel (31), social worker in a hospital team:

'I was so upset when this consultant treated me like a skivvy in a multi-disciplinary meeting of all places, expecting me to do what *he* thought was best for the patient, without any consultation about their home or social circumstances. Fortunately I spoke to him afterwards and he at least had the grace to listen to my point of view. And to my amazement I got him to agree to postpone the discharge until we had completed our assessments. I do seriously worry, though, that some senior professionals regard us from another profession as a dogsbody to be at their beck and call.'

# INTERVIEWING CHILDREN

This whole book, in some way, deals with the basic skills of interviewing. From the moment you welcome someone for the first time, to how you bring the meeting to a close; from how you ask questions and gather information, to how your non-verbal communication makes an impact – all of these communication skills are at the heart of interviewing. There are nevertheless some specific issues involved in interviewing children which deserve special attention.

Social workers, family mediators, doctors, health visitors, nurses, police officers and probation officers: these and many other professionals will, from time to time, be required to interview children formally, and it is of crucial importance that the careful guidelines for good practice are scrupulously followed. This is particularly important where there are cases of child abuse to be investigated. *Working Together to Safeguard Children* (DCSF, 2013) insists that all assessments should be child-centred, stating that 'Initial discussions with the child should be conducted in a way that minimizes distress to them and maximizes the likelihood that they will provide accurate and complete information, avoiding leading or suggestive questions' (2013: 30). This means that however complex the interviewing process may be with adults, when children are involved there are additional layers of complexity that must be taken into account.

It is essential at this point to highlight the seminal work of Eileen Munro (2011) in her review of child protection issues, and her proposal to enable professionals to make the best judgements to help children, young people and families. Her emphasis is upon professional expertise that prioritises the safety and welfare of children, and seeks to avoid too bureaucratic an approach. You must engage thoroughly not only with this report, so that you can understand better how previous well-intentioned reforms have not delivered the expected level of improvements, but also with key legislation such as the United Nations Convention on the Rights of the Child (UNICEF, 1990) and the Human Rights Act 1998. These provide the context for much of your work.

The worrying background to this discussion, with the many examples of social workers, police officers and paediatric consultants not always communicating effectively together, has led to a difficult climate in which to work with children. Professional workers find themselves constantly looking over their shoulders, hoping they 'don't get it wrong – again', and many colleagues in the field of children's work report high levels of stress and anxiety as they seek to fulfil their obligations and responsibilities.

The challenging climate for this work should not blind you, however, to its crucial importance. One of the hallmarks of a civilised, caring society is the way in which vulnerable people are regarded and respected, and the ways in which children and young people are cherished, valued and encouraged to live their lives to their fullest potential to help them achieve the five positive outcomes identified in *Every Child Matters* (DfES, 2004). Anyone who exploits or abuses children is not only damaging the individual child, they are also undermining the basic societal values that cherish children and their place in society. The duty – and privilege – of protecting and safeguarding children is therefore of paramount importance, and just because there are inherent difficulties in the task does not mean we should ever flinch from it.

## Activity

Think about your role as a worker with children. What are the good and positive aspects of this work? What are the negative aspects of it, or the 'downsides' of the work? When you have completed this list, use it as a basis for discussion with your colleagues, supervisor or practice educator. This will help you gain a better picture not only of the work itself, but also of how you are approaching it, what your strengths are and the aspects of the work that make you feel nervous or inadequate.

When you think about your work with children, it is important not to begin with the children, but with yourself as a worker. This involves not only an awareness of the skills you will need to undertake the work, but also a heightened awareness of yourself and how you come across to others. It is, admittedly, extremely difficult to see yourself 'through a child's or young person's eyes', but some attempt must be made as part of your commitment to anti-discriminatory practice and to being a reflective practitioner. If a child has had their trust in adults undermined or destroyed, it is hardly surprising that they may regard you with some suspicion simply because you are an adult, however different you may be from the adult who has betrayed their trust. You will be seen as a powerful adult, and you will need to practise the communication skills of establishing trust before any meaningful work can be undertaken.

If you are honest, your work with children, or at least your attitude towards it, may be determined, to some extent at least, by your own experience of childhood, and perhaps your own experience of being a parent or grandparent. There are also many excellent social workers and other professionals working with children who themselves have been previous victims of abuse. But they have subsequently sought appropriate help to ensure that these experiences do not get in the way of their work, but rather deepen their motivation to protect others from similar harm.

Some adults find young people a bit 'scary', especially when they enter their teenage years: they find their 'grunt-laden apathy' or their boundary-testing exuberance too hot to handle. Others, by contrast, exult in the freshness, enthusiasm and uncertainties of youth, and get a huge 'buzz' from working with young people. Furthermore, individuals' experiences of their school days are as varied as they could possibly be, and yours too will have had some impact upon how you view children and young people currently going through a school education.

# Activity

The previous paragraph touched on different attitudes to children and young people, and how your experiences may impact upon your approach. This Activity is intended to help you 'locate yourself' as a worker, and to help you understand yourself a bit better. Make two lists on a piece of paper: in the first list note down all the positive experiences and memories of being a child and a young person that you can recall; the second is a list of all the negative, difficult and painful memories and experiences you can recall. Be as honest as you can, and try not to rush the exercise. When you have completed it, think about what the implications are for you in your work with children and young people. It would be good to share this list with someone you can trust, and if you are a student in training it would be good to use this as a basis for a supervision session looking at your values and how you are approaching this kind of work. Keep the list safe – you may find you want to add to it as time goes by. Remember, the most important thing you bring to your work is yourself, and how you come across to people will determine to a great extent how effective you can be as a worker.

People of all ages need to know that they are accepted and valued; they deserve to receive an anti-discriminatory service, and to feel that they are included in what is being done in a real partnership. Just because people are young in years does not mean that these core communication skills are any less relevant. Children and young people welcome positive feedback just as anyone else does, and will thrive on an empowering approach. The challenges of diversity remain just as acute: children and young people from minority ethnic groups, or who have learning difficulties or some experience of disability, need workers who are aware of the wider cultural and societal aspects of discrimination and oppression, and who can incorporate these perspectives appropriately into their practice. In short, children and young people deserve the same 'gold standard' service as anyone else in the community: anything less is a betrayal of the best practice commitment all people-workers need to uphold.

Curran et al. (2013: 40) provide a useful list of the communication skills necessary for the safeguarding and promoting of the welfare of the child. These include:

- Establishing rapport and respectful, trusting relationships with children, young people and those caring for them.
- Understanding what is meant by safeguarding and the different ways in which children and young people can be harmed (including by other children, young people and adults through the Internet).
- Making considered judgements about how to safeguard and promote a child or young person's welfare, and, where appropriate, consulting with the child, young person, parent or carer to inform your thinking.
- Giving the child or young person the opportunity to participate in decisions affecting them – appropriate to their age and ability – and taking their wishes and feelings into account.
- Understanding the key role of parents and carers in safeguarding and promoting children and young people's welfare and involving them accordingly, while recognising factors that can affect parenting and increase the risk of abuse (e.g. domestic violence).

- Understanding that signs of abuse can be subtle and can be expressed in play, artwork and in the way children and young people approach relationships with other children and/or adults.
- Making considered judgements about how to act to safeguard and promote a child or young person's welfare.
- Being able to use clear language to communicate information unambiguously to others, including children, young people, their families and carers.
- Listening carefully to what is said and checking understanding.

You need, in short, to take time to consider the needs of each individual child. This will assist you in undertaking the relevant preparatory assessment of how best to encourage positive communication between you.

There is one further caveat, especially when multi-agency work is being undertaken. Each agency tends to collect its own information when meeting with the child and their family, but as Pestana cautions,

> children say that the one thing they get 'fed-up' with is having continually to repeat their story to professional workers. There is a danger here that children may become complacent and not share all relevant information due to feeling they are having to repeat themselves. (Personal communication)

Interprofessional exchange of information, and careful preparation beforehand, therefore, are increasingly important.

## Group exercise

With the help of your tutor or supervisor, spend some time working through the list of communication skills given above, and identify those areas where you feel you would need particular help and support in being able to achieve a successful outcome. You may find it helpful to have a particular example in mind of some work you have done to help you focus on these issues.

## COMPLEX NEEDS

Working with disabled children, and children with complex needs, increases the range of communication skills you will need. In whatever professional capacity you work, there is a network of support and supervision to help you practise and gain competence in using the appropriate communication skills. You should not be thrown in at the deep end or left to flounder; there is considerable professional expertise upon which you can draw to develop your own skills. You also need to become fully aware of the implications of the Children and Families Act 2014 and how it affects disabled children and their families.

It will be clear to you that when it comes to definitions, the notion of complex needs is very wide ranging, but it generally refers to children who have more than one impairment, or who have major healthcare needs such as life-limiting conditions, and those who have developed an impairment as a result of maltreatment or abuse. The communication skills you will need to develop, therefore, must be appropriate to the specific needs of the individual child. There is always a danger of compartmentalising such needs, of course, and you are advised to consult specialist literature and relevant colleagues to help you work with particular children with complex needs.

It is important, however, that you now return to the point made at the outset of this discussion. You must be aware of the impact of such issues upon you, your attitudes, values and approach. Some children with complex needs present the worker with particular challenges, especially if there is physical disfigurement, or uncoordinated speech or physical movement. You should be aware of the impact of your non-verbal communication towards the young person and the family; if you feel an element of revulsion (this is a strong word to use, but there is no point in 'pussyfooting' around such issues, which can provoke strong reactions in some people), then this will communicate itself very clearly to them. It is of vital importance, therefore, that you examine your own value base and your own attitudes in advance of such work, so that you can ensure that you provide the level of acceptance, respect and care that the person has every right to receive from you. This is part of what is meant by being a reflective practitioner.

You will have noticed throughout this entire discussion that you and your communication skills are being put in the spotlight far more than the particular child or young person who has complex needs. This is not to minimise the child's needs or the quality of complex services that may be necessary – far from it. But it does emphasise your importance as the worker, *what* you are communicating and *how* you are communicating. If you can get that right, the other things will follow, given appropriate support, advice, training and guidance. You will find the Community Care Inform website with its online resources for social workers extremely helpful in this regard (www.ccinform.co.uk).

## DEALING WITH HARM

When there is information and evidence to suggest that a child has suffered significant harm, a joint investigation with the police and a social worker who has received specific training will be undertaken under Section 47 of the Children Act 1989. Achieving best evidence (ABE) interviews are usually undertaken in a comfortable location, and not a police station environment. It is important that a child can feel relatively at ease, so that they feel able to share information regarding their experience.

ABE interviews are generally led by the police for the criminal investigation perspective. However, 'the decision as to who leads the interview should depend on who is able to establish the best rapport with the child' (Ministry of Justice, 2011). It is important to recognise, therefore, that sometimes as a social worker you may already know the child, and may have a good relationship with them, as well as a level of understanding of the child's previous 'lived experiences'. On other occasions, however, this could be their first involvement with you and therefore the building blocks of this relationship will start from the very beginning. This core social work skill is essential, however challenging it might be. Distress needs to be minimised, so that the child feels respected, reassured and listened to, otherwise they will not feel able to engage with you.

The ABE interview can 'inform enquiries regarding significant harm under Section 47 of The Children Act 1989 and any subsequent actions to safeguard and promote the child's welfare, and in some cases, the welfare of other children' (Ministry of Justice, 2011).

ABE interviews are undertaken using TED questions (Tell, Explain, Describe), which use open-ended questioning to ask a child to: Tell – what happened; Explain it – which can be encouraged further by asking 'and then what happened?'; and then Describe it – which gathers detail to substantiate the information gathered. This simple but effective tool will help you gain detailed information in an open-ended way that helps the child tell their story to the best effect.

'Getting it right' when working with children who have experienced harm is never easy. You will find it demanding, both professionally and personally, on your skills and values, and also with your capacity to work collegially with other professionals, but if you can help to keep a child safe then that is all that matters.

## UNACCOMPANIED ASYLUM-SEEKING CHILDREN

Unaccompanied asylum-seeking children (UASC) is an area of work that has become increasingly significant in recent years. The core skills you will use will be the same, but there are some specific challenges to this work that deserve mention. For example, a female social worker may encounter different cultural expectations in children whose cultural norms have been significantly different in their country of origin. As a female you may be considered 'less able' and 'not to be respected', especially if there is uncertainty and unfamiliarity with what a social worker's role involves.

It is essential that UASC are offered an interpreter who not only speaks the same language, but if possible can also communicate using the same dialect. The child should feel comfortable with their interpreter and recognise that they can use this support to convey any difficulties, distress or frustrations they may feel. You will need also to recognise that if a female child has suffered abuse, you may need to ensure that there is a female interpreter available to work with them.

As a social worker you will need to maintain a professional balance in your relationship with UASC. Although this may take time, if you can develop a trusting, partnership-working relationship you will not only be able to support them but also encourage them to nurture their resilience and capacity to take their own decisions.

## CARERS AND YOUNG CARERS

In the discussion on empowerment, resilience and a strengths perspective, you were encouraged always to think about the capacity people have to tackle problems creatively, and to find ways of fostering their resilience and inner strength in times of difficulty or crisis. Perhaps nowhere are these particular attributes more clearly evident than in the unsung army of carers, both young and old, who selflessly devote time, energy, love and attention to looking after a parent, relative or child. For young carers, this will take place alongside all the other things they have to do, such as attending school and having something of a social life as well. To work with carers is a humbling privilege, and will bring into sharp focus your values and communication skills. Any hint of being patronising or condescending will be seen through quickly, but a commitment to working in respectful partnership will be welcomed.

## Group exercise

How aware are you and your team of the work done by carers and young carers in your area? Find out about your local carers' associations, what they offer, and what level of support and encouragement they need in order to continue with their important work, and share this with your group. With the help of your tutor or supervisor, discuss the implications for your own practice.

## FINAL THOUGHTS

Anyone working with children and young people will be aware of the vast literature that now exists to encourage, support and guide workers in this important field, both for generic working and for the delivery of more specialist services. A few of these are listed below, but within your agency you will have access to much more, including recent policy developments. These are valuable resources: do use them.

## REFERENCES AND FURTHER READING

Barker, R. (ed.) (2008) *Making Sense of Every Child Matters: Multi-professional Practice Guidance*. Bristol: Policy Press.

Bomber, L.M. (2007) *Inside I'm Hurting: Practical Strategies for Supporting Children with Attachment Difficulties in Schools*. London: Worth.

Children and Families Act (2014) Available at https://b.barnardos.org.uk/factsheet_1_-_introduction_-_final.pdf (accessed 22/11/19).

Curran, S., Harrison, R. and Mackinnon, D. (2013) *Working with Young People*, 2nd edition. London: Open University/Sage.

Department for Children, Schools and Families (DCSF) (2013) *Working Together to Safeguard Children: A Guide to Interagency Working to Safeguard and Promote the Welfare of Children*. Nottingham: DCSF Publications.

Department for Education and Skills (DfES) (2004) *Every Child Matters*. London: DfES.

Human Rights Act (1998). Available at: www.legislation.gov.uk/ukpga/1998/42/contents (accessed 15/10/19).

Jowitt, M. and O'Loughlin, S. (2016) *Social Work with Children and Families*, 4th edition. Exeter: Learning Matters.

Lefevre, M. (2018) *Communicating with Children and Young People: Making a Difference*, 2nd edition. Bristol: Policy Press.

Milner, J. and Bateman, J. (2011) *Working with Children and Teenagers using Solution Focused Approaches: Enabling Children to Overcome Challenges and Achieve their Potential.* London: Jessica Kingsley.

Ministry of Justice (2011) 'Achieving best evidence in criminal proceedings'. Available at www.cps.gov.uk/sites/default/files/documents/legal_guidance/best_evidence_in_criminal_proceedings.pdf (accessed 21/10/2019).

Munro, E. (2011) *Munro Review of Child Protection: A Final Report – A Child-Centred System.* London: Department of Education.

Tait, A. and Wosu, H. (2013) *Direct Work with Vulnerable Children: Playful Activities and Strategies for Communication.* London: Jessica Kingsley.

UNICEF (1990) United Nations Convention on the Rights of the Child (1989). London: UNICEF. Available at https://downloads.unicef.org.uk/wp-content/uploads/2010/05/UNCRC_united_nations_convention_on_the_rights_of_the_child.pdf?_ga=2.264748107.575847088.1571149510-1835864007.1571149510 (accessed 15/10/19).

Web resource

Community Care Inform, Decision-making essential resources – www.ccinform.co.uk (accessed 11/09/19)

**RELATED CONCEPTS** acceptance; anti-discriminatory practice; assessment; empowerment; interpreters; interprofessional collaboration; reflective practice; resilience and a strengths perspective

**ENGAGING WITH THE PCF** critical reflection; diversity; skills and interventions; professionalism; values and ethics

**ENGAGING WITH THE NMC CODE** prioritise people; preserve safety

Service user snippet

Benjamin (13), in foster care:

'I hate talking with grown-ups – it's vile – but Lynsey is different – OK she's old, but at least she gets down on the floor to talk with me.'

# LABYRINTHS

One of the communication skills that people-workers need to develop is the exploration of various artefacts that can facilitate communication both for themselves and for those they are seeking to help. Ecomaps and genograms are two examples of this. Another example is the increasing use of labyrinths both as a stress-busting activity and also as a powerful aid to communication and creativity.

As Figure 6 shows, a labyrinth is a single pathway that twists and turns until it reaches a central point. This journey towards the centre – whether undertaken on a large-scale labyrinth on which you can actually walk, or on a smaller version that you can trace with a finger on a wooden or sketched version – allows you to focus your thoughts or to empty your mind of what may be worrying you. There is something about the gentle rhythm of following the path that can be relaxing. It can also be a metaphor for the twists and turns of our life, especially when we are not at all sure about the direction we are heading in or the goal we are seeking to attain.

A labyrinth is a neutral space in that it leaves it up to whoever is using or walking it to decide what they wish to gain from it. For some it is an opportunity for a short time of quiet reflection and relaxation as they trace the pathway to the centre and back again. Others will want to bring a particular problem or challenge to their walk and hope that by focusing upon it during their walk they will gain greater clarity or insight. Sometimes it can be a therapeutic activity whereby a particular

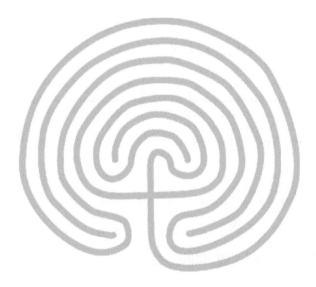

**Figure 6**   Hand-drawn labyrinth

burden or guilt, shame, abuse or loss can be taken to the centre point and symbolically left there. For some for whom faith is important it can be a prayer mat and an opportunity to pray for themselves or for others.

---

## Activity

See if there is a full-size labyrinth near you (see www.labyrinthlocator.com) that you can visit and walk it. Alternatively, download one from the website www.labyrinthsociety.org and give it a go!

---

## Group exercise

With the help of your tutor or supervisor, arrange a group session to create your own temporary full-size labyrinth (Sellers and Moss, 2016: 31ff). As well as being an enjoyable group exercise it will provide an opportunity for you to walk it as a group and to share your thoughts and reflections afterwards.

## FINAL THOUGHTS

As with other artefacts, it is up to you how you wish to make use of it, for yourself or with someone you are seeking to help and support. If you feel confident enough, do try using a hand-drawn labyrinth or one you can download from the Web. There is no guaranteed outcome, but there is a developing body of evidence which talks about the calming 'labyrinth effect' on people's lives and the creative opportunities it can offer as an aid to communication at a deep level.

 ## REFERENCES AND FURTHER READING

Doel, M. (2017) *Social Work in 40 Objects (and More)*. Lichfield: Kirwin Maclean Associates.
Sellers, J. and Moss, B. (2016) *Learning with the Labyrinth: Creating Reflective Space in Higher Education*. Basingstoke: Palgrave Macmillan. (*Note*: This book provides a fascinating insight and introduction to labyrinths and their use in a range of academic and professional disciplines, including several people-work professions.)

**RELATED CONCEPTS** ecomaps; genograms; professionalism; reflective practice

**ENGAGING WITH THE PCF** critical reflection and analysis

**ENGAGING WITH THE NMC CODE** practise effectively; promote professionalism and trust

### Service user snippet

Amy, student:

'The walk was profound. It sparked new ideas, showed me another perspective about others ... we are all different on a different path but we all want to get to the centre. It helped to release my judgment.' (Cited in Sellers and Moss, 2016: 145)

# LEARNING DIFFICULTIES

To discuss learning difficulties in a book about communication skills immediately invites disquiet by assuming a 'them and us' mentality, whereby we mistakenly attribute all sorts of communication 'problems' to one group of people who somehow are not as 'fortunate' as others. Terminology is revealing. The term 'learning difficulty' is often preferred because it conveys the message that certain things about living, loving, surviving and succeeding are difficult. Everyone can identify to some extent with that statement!

Some prefer the term 'learning disabilities' or more recently 'intellectual disabilities'. This runs the risk of course of straying into a medicalised, 'sickness' model rather than celebrating (as we would prefer) the social model of disability, with its emphasis upon how societal attitudes shape the way people are treated and regarded. Instead of appreciating each individual's strengths and challenges, we often lump people together into homogeneous groups in very discriminatory and oppressive ways, assuming that *one size fits all* when it comes to communication and interaction. Even professional people-workers can sometimes fall into this trap. The language we use therefore is really important and powerful. As Golding and Moss argue,

> even language that started life as 'neutral' can become imbued with meaning and become unacceptable. It is important to be mindful about the effects of labels and to ensure that people have choice about how they are described. (2019: 17)

The first point to stress, therefore, is the value base that underpins all people-work. The importance of affording acceptance, dignity, respect and value to each and every human being is a non-negotiable principle. The communication skills, both verbal and non-verbal, that both embody and reflect these principles should be the same for everyone, no matter what additional labels they may be given. The White Paper *Valuing People* (DH, 2001) sought to embody and 'flesh out' what a value-based approach to working with people with learning difficulties would look like.

A second introductory and underpinning point stresses the talents, gifts, creative abilities and resilience that we believe everyone has to a greater or lesser extent. Therefore, the basic principles of partnership working, empowerment, and the clutch of issues that are raised by an awareness of people's spirituality, are not only relevant but crucial to our approach. We must always be open to being caught by surprise when another person's talents burst forth in unexpected ways and places.

To our shame we often do not expect people with learning difficulties to surprise us. Williams (2013: 128) reminds us that,

> There are people so described who have written poetry and books, become artists and performers, given talks at conferences, have played a valuable role in teaching professionals, have acted as consultants on government policy and so on.

The third point to make is that we often talk as if any problems and difficulties lie with the other person, not ourselves. But time and again, the real problem may lie with us, and our inability to understand, accept and empathise. Just as it always takes two to tango, it takes two to communicate; and if we are putting up barriers, then no wonder communication is difficult.

## Activity

Spend some time reflecting on the three introductory points made above, and relate them to someone with learning difficulties whom you know. Have you discovered in yourself the temptation to play down these core values in your dealings with them? What do you feel are the biggest issues for you in seeking to establish meaningful and effective communication with people with learning difficulties? For a more general appreciation of some of the issues raised here, look at Mencap's (2007) important report *Death by Indifference*.

If you have completed this exercise honestly, a number of reactions may have been triggered. Perhaps you have identified some learning difficulty within yourself. Most, if not all, of us struggle to learn certain skills, or to express ourselves clearly, and a realistic awareness of this, tinged with a degree of humility, can help to reinforce the bonds of common humanity between us and those with whom we are called to work with in our professional people-work roles.

Another reaction may be elicited by certain physical characteristics in others that you may find disturbing. The key issue here is captured in the words *that you may find disturbing*. This indicates that the problem, if indeed there is a problem, lies with you and your inability or unwillingness to celebrate diversity. Other people's differences will impact upon you and how you relate to them. As the discussion on non-verbal communication reveals, these deep feelings will communicate themselves to others very easily. If you feel embarrassed or disgusted, that will communicate itself to the other person, and will counteract any words you use to convey your professional value base of acceptance and respect. The importance of reflective practice, therefore, cannot be underestimated.

Key points to bear in mind when seeking to communicate with someone with learning difficulties include:

- Remember that the other person is the 'expert' and will know what works best; each person is unique.
- Key principles of acceptance, dignity, respect and working in partnership must always be central to your approach.
- Your own non-verbal communication skills will be particularly important.
- Be reflective in trying to identify and then remove barriers you are putting up that get in the way of effective communication.
- A trusting relationship is crucial; however mechanistic a 'system' such as Makaton may seem, it is the quality of your relationship that is all-important.
- Explore ways of helping the other person to 'play to their strengths'.
- Work in partnership with others who may know the other person far better than you do.
- Ensure that you are aware of the NHS Accessible Information Standard and that your own practice meets these requirements (www.england.nhs.uk/accessibleinfo).

---

### Group exercise

With the help of your tutor or supervisor, explore the NHS England 2016 (revised 2017) Accessible Information Standard. What are the implications for your own practice? What challenges does this Standard pose for your organisations?

---

## SOME SPECIALIST TECHNIQUES

Within this overall framework of values that underpin your professional practice, there are some communication skills, however, that are particularly appropriate to use with people with very severe impairments. Two systems are often found to be helpful: Makaton and Signalong, which are simplified variations of British Sign Language, which is the principal and very fluent first language of the Deaf community. Another approach is the use of the Widgit system that enables written words to be turned into visual symbols. These systems can be enormously helpful aids to communication, but clearly they need a mutual familiarity for them to be effective, along with a sensitive, patient approach by the worker (for further details of these three systems, see www.makaton.org, www.signalong.org.uk and www.widgit.com).

There is a temptation, however, to shoehorn everyone into a handful of communication 'techniques', and to assume that one size fits all. The real communication skill lies in seeking out what is most effective for each individual. Some people, for example, thrive on the possibilities of new electronic technologies that can enable people who previously had been unable to express themselves clearly to others, to begin to pour their self-expression onto the screen. 'Facilitated communication', whereby someone guides and supports the other person to help them write and spell words, has also had some dramatic creative results (see Williams, 2013: 128, for some examples).

## FINAL THOUGHTS

The stories you hear about the ways in which people with learning difficulties are sometimes treated – stories of abuse; of not being treated with respect and dignity in supported accommodation, residential settings or in hospital; or being refused entry to restaurants, for example – will remind you that underlying all communication skills is your value base. Until you get that right, you will not be able to really communicate appropriately with another human being, nor treat them with dignity and respect, and as valued human beings.

## REFERENCES AND FURTHER READING

Department of Health (DH) (2001) *Valuing People: A New Strategy for Learning Disability for the 21st Century*, Cm 5086. London: Department of Health.
Golding, L. and Moss, J. (2019) *How to Become a Clinical Psychologist*. Abingdon: Routledge.
Mencap (2007) *Death by Indifference*. London: Mencap. Available at www.mencap.org.uk/sites/default/files/2016-06/DBIreport.pdf (accessed 15/10/19).
Mencap (2012) *Death by Indifference: 74 Deaths and Counting – A Progress Report 5 Years On*. London: Mencap. Available at www.mencap.org.uk/sites/default/files/2016-08/Death%20by%20Indifference%20-%2074%20deaths%20and%20counting.pdf (accessed 15/10/19).
NHS England (2016) 'Accessible information standard'. Available at www.england.nhs.uk/accessibleinfo (accessed 21/10/19).
Swinton, J. (2002) 'Spirituality and the lives of people with learning disabilities', *The Tizard Learning Disability Review*, 7 (4): 29–35.
Williams, P. (2013) *Social Work with People with Learning Difficulties*, 3rd edition. Exeter: Learning Matters. (*Note*: this book has much to offer people-workers from other disciplines.)
Woodcock Ross, J. (2016) *Specialist Communication Skills for Social Workers: Developing Professional Capability*, 2nd edition. Basingstoke: Palgrave Macmillan.

### Web resources

Makaton, language programme – www.makaton.org (accessed 11/09/19)
Sing Along, for the under-5s – www.singalong.org.uk (accessed 11/09/19)
Widgit, symbols and software titles to aid communication – www.widgit.com (accessed 11/09/19)

**RELATED CONCEPTS** active listening; non-verbal communication; reflective practice; spirituality

**ENGAGING WITH THE PCF** critical reflection and analysis; diversity; skills and interventions; values and ethics

**ENGAGING WITH THE NMC CODE** prioritise people; preserve safety

## Service user snippet

Leon (32), living in sheltered accommodation:

'I really like my worker – he's called Brian – he never seems to be in a rush – I like him a lot. He treats me like a grown up.'

# LOSS

The experience of loss is a common theme in people-work: dealing with loss is a cost of being human. It is, therefore, important that people-workers develop the communication skills to be able to work sensitively and appropriately with people who are experiencing loss.

## Activity

Jot down as many examples of loss, minor and major, as you can. Check that you have covered a wide age range in your list – loss can and does happen at any age. Keep this list beside you as you work through this discussion.

The list you have just compiled may well grow in length the more you think about it. You have probably included some major losses such as divorce, unemployment, ill health and bereavement, as well as a wide variety of seemingly less significant losses, like losing your purse or wallet or a favourite item of clothing. Some losses are difficult to define, such as the loss of faith or confidence, while others may be too painful to share with other people.

In thinking about the communication skills needed to work with people experiencing loss, it is important to acknowledge that perhaps more than any other topic, this can deeply affect us as workers. The experience of loss is so pervasive: how we have dealt with our own losses will have some impact upon how we respond to others going through a similar experience. For example:

- If you have not fully grieved over the loss of someone close to you, you may find that working with someone recently and painfully bereaved can trigger painful memories within you which you desperately want to ignore or avoid.
- If you have had a difficult or painful experience of divorce within your own family, you may find working with couples with children who are separating extremely upsetting.
- If your health has deteriorated or you have suddenly become disabled in some way, this may have an impact upon your self-image and the confidence you have when dealing with others.
- If, in the past, you have been 'given the sack' from a job and are trying to work with a person in a similar situation, you may find yourself strongly identifying with them and assuming that what was true for you will be true for them. You

may find yourself urging them to pursue a course of action that seems right to you, based on your experience, but which may not be right for them.

- If your own experiences of loss are difficult and painful, you may find yourself steering conversations and interviews away from this topic in order to make the interview more manageable and comfortable for you, even if the other person really needs to discuss it.

These examples illustrate how a traumatic experience may negatively affect your working relationship with others. By contrast, however, if you have yourself been 'through the prickly hedge of grief and loss', and have benefitted from loving support and TLC, then you could have less 'baggage' to get in the way of your work with others going through similar experiences.

This emphasis upon our experience of loss as workers is important, because inevitably we will be communicating to the other person non-verbally a number of messages which they will pick up on even more quickly because of the rawness and sensitivity of their own feelings. So, if you are feeling awkward, embarrassed, tense, agitated or scared, this will communicate itself to the other person, who will perhaps think twice before opening up about how they are really feeling. If, on the other hand, you can convey warmth, acceptance, a sense of stillness and a willingness to be with the other person, then it is likely that they will receive the message that it is safe to talk to you, because somehow, just somehow, you may understand.

In other words, how we deal with our own losses will determine to a large extent how we deal with others and their loss.

The second main area for us as people-workers to grasp when developing our communication skills when responding to loss is the importance of a sound theoretical perspective to help us – and the other person – understand what they are going through. There are several dimensions to this:

1   The person experiencing the loss is the only one who can say how intense their feelings are. What may appear as a minor loss to the worker (the death of a pet budgerigar, for example), may be a major loss to the older person who had been living alone unable to get out and about, and for whom the budgie was a real source of comfort and company, and even perhaps a reason to keep going. If the worker seeks to minimise the impact of a loss, this could be resented by the other person, who will immediately feel that the worker simply does not understand.

2   Comforting words are often not comforting. Workers can easily fall into the trap of thinking that there is a word for every occasion, and seek to offer comfort with what are often no more than platitudes. For example:

'You'll soon get over it.'
'There are plenty of other fish in the sea.'
'You'll be OK, I promise.'
'There are plenty of others worse off than you.'
'Try to pull yourself together.'
'Why don't you take up a hobby, get out and meet people.'

3   There is, of course, a tiny germ of truth lurking in each of these statements, but they rarely help: they tell us more about the worker's needs and where the

worker is coming from rather than where the other person is currently standing. At best, they are well meaning; at worst, they are a banal 'whistling in the dark' by a bemused worker who does not know how to communicate with someone experiencing loss.

4    There is no automatic process for dealing with grief and loss. Many people-workers have been brought up on the seminal work by Elizabeth Kubler Ross (1969), who, with others, talked about the stages of grief through which people need to pass before reaching the final point of acceptance. Her work with dying people revealed some of the profound feelings that loss provokes: shock, anger, denial, despair. Anyone who has experienced a profound loss will identify with these feelings, and know how powerful they can be. What has been less helpful is the way in which some people-workers have used the stages model almost to predict the journey through grief, and to regard the model as being prescriptive. A lot of contemporary theorists have helped us move towards a more complex and realistic understanding of how people respond to grief and loss, by reminding us that everyone's journey is unique and that each of us chooses, consciously or otherwise, how we will handle such matters. Two contemporary approaches may be of particular help to people-workers in general.

- Neimeyer (2001) talks about meaning reconstruction, which emphasises that it is the person who is experiencing the grief and loss who knows the *meaning* of that loss, and more importantly how new meanings will need to be created if life is to go on in any meaningful way in the future. This journey towards new meanings may be never-ending, of course, but the search for them is critical.
- The 'dual process' model of Stroebe and Schutt (1999) talks of two orientations when we experience loss: the past and the present/future. The journey of grief will see people moving in and out of these two orientations, sometimes many times in a day, as they are at one time overwhelmed by the loss, and at other times facing the daily tasks that have to be undertaken, while looking ahead. As time goes by, they will spend less and less time in the past orientation, but it will never go away, and is likely to be re-stimulated at key moments in the year, such as anniversaries, or by key moments such as hearing a particular tune or going to a particular place.

This is but a quick snapshot of some of the theoretical perspectives which are enriching our understanding of grief and loss, and you are encouraged to explore these in greater depth, together with other perspectives, through the further reading listed below. The perspectives that have been covered, however, are sufficient to illustrate some of the main communication skills necessary when working with people who are experiencing loss:

- *Be aware of your non-verbal communication*: Be open, accepting and unhurried in your approach – do not sit with arms crossed or look as if you have chewed a wasp; avoid barrier gestures; watch with smiling eyes and a subtle, warm but not cheery smile.

- *Ask – don't tell*: Invite the person to say how they are feeling, and what their loss means to them. Encourage them to talk about their loss if they wish.
- *Explain but don't predict*: Your grasp of theoretical perspectives and how people often react to serious loss can be helpful to others if handled sensitively. The dual process model, for example, can be explained simply to reassure people that they will ebb and flow in their feelings, probably for quite a long time, and this is not something to be unduly worried about. The more precious something or someone has been to them, the more acute and long-lasting the reactions to the loss will be. Maybe they will never ever fully 'get over' the loss or come to terms with it: in such situations, their future may be about learning to surround the gaping hole in their lives with various people and activities, knowing full well that the hole will never close. The thing to avoid is predicting how people will react: we are all different and we cannot predict when or how people will deal with their loss. If, for example, as sometimes happens, workers slavishly follow the stages model and try to reassure people that after such and such a stage things will improve, this could be disheartening for the person if this is not what happens. They may feel that they are doing something wrong when things do not follow the pattern they have been led to expect. Again, the reassurance lies in explaining to people that we all do things differently, and that getting it right for them is the crucial thing. Certain feelings are common: a loss of energy or interest is to be expected; physical symptoms such as backache can sometimes be experienced. Some people feel they are in a dark tunnel that has no end to it. Again, tempting though it is to try to predict how soon these feelings will abate, we cannot do this with any integrity: after all, we could be very wrong in our predictions. Instead, finding ways of empathising with their pain, fear and discomfort is far more helpful in the long run.
- *Share their journey – don't make it your own*: Empathy is crucial. People do not want to hear about your journey or what did or did not work for you, but to have someone who will listen in a caring non-judgemental way, to help them feel at least to a small extent that they are not as totally alone as they had feared. You can never fully understand or get inside another person's experience of loss, or what it means to them, but if you make the attempt it can prove to be very supportive. However, you must not make the other person's burden your own, or get so embroiled in their difficulties that you lose your objectivity and professional distance. This is why an awareness of your own losses is so important: if the other person's loss triggers off painful deep-seated feelings within you, then you begin to lose your professional perspective and become part of the problem rather than providing support to the person on their journey.
- *Explore – don't interrogate*: The style you adopt in talking with someone experiencing loss is all-important. Too vigorous, insensitive or persistent questioning will likely make someone 'close down' and become resentful that their personal space is being invaded. You can, however, begin to explore with the person how they think they will begin to face and re-shape their future, and begin to engage with the meaning of the reconstruction that will soon be necessary, to a greater or lesser extent. But if you push too hard and give the impression that you are expecting the other person to come up with clear-cut

answers and strategies, then you are likely to undermine what little confidence they have clung onto.

- *Religious faith and spirituality*: The issue of people's religious faith, or their more general spirituality which shapes their world view, is another issue that needs to be explored in an open, sensitive way. In all cases, as the worker you must ensure that whatever the world view to which you personally subscribe, it is the other person's world view that is important and the extent to which it proves satisfying and helpful to them in moments of crisis and loss.

## Group exercise

With the help of your tutor or supervisor, discuss your reactions to and your feelings about the main points mentioned above, paying particular attention to 'explore, don't interrogate', the issues about religious faith, and how to respond if a service user or patient asks you about your own losses or your own world view.

## FINAL THOUGHTS

Because loss is such a pervasive experience, it is inevitable that it will directly impinge upon your practice. Your generic communication skills will stand you in good stead to ensure that the person feels valued and supported. However, there may well be situations where the other person seems so deeply immersed, even trapped, in their feelings of loss, pain and disempowerment that you realise that they need more specific professional help than you are able to provide. In such situations, you need to know what range of local services, including bereavement counselling, is available, and to find sensitive ways of referring people to these services without seeming to reject them. It is important that you feel able to use the skills guidelines we have suggested here, but it is also vital that you know your limitations and do not try to swim in waters that are far too deep for you to navigate successfully and professionally.

## REFERENCES AND FURTHER READING

Currer, C. (2007) *Loss and Social Work: Transforming Social Work Practice*. Exeter: Learning Matters.

Holloway, M. (2007) *Negotiating Death in Contemporary Health and Social Care*. Bristol: Policy Press.

Holloway, M. and Moss, B. (2010) *Spirituality and Social Work*. Basingstoke: Palgrave Macmillan.

Kubler Ross, E. (1969) *On Death and Dying*. New York: Palgrave Macmillan.

Neimeyer, R. (2001) *Meaning Reconstruction and the Meaning of Loss*. Washington, DC: American Psychological Association.

Stroebe, M. and Schutt, M. (1999) 'The dual process model of coping with bereavement: rationale and description', *Death Studies*, 23 (3): 197–224.

Thompson, N. (2012) *Grief and its Challenges*. Basingstoke: Palgrave Macmillan.

**RELATED CONCEPTS** active listening; barrier gestures; empathy; non-verbal communication; religion; empowerment, resilience and a strengths perspective; spirituality

**ENGAGING WITH THE PCF** critical reflection and analysis; knowledge; professionalism; skills and interventions; values and ethics

**ENGAGING WITH THE NMC CODE** prioritise people; practise effectively

### Service user snippet

Shirley (68), bereaved relative in an oncology ward:

'It was such a relief just to talk about how I felt when Stan was taken from us so suddenly. I felt numb – my world had come to an end, and even my faith was shaken. But Liz just listened, and it was like being wrapped in a lovely warm blanket.'

# MEDIATION SKILLS

Mediation, as a practice discipline, is a very skilled process whereby a person 'in the middle' seeks to facilitate a creative, acceptable outcome for two people who are in dispute and conflict with each other. The person in the middle – the mediator – seeks impartially to create an environment of mutual respect to enable the disputants to come to some level of agreement, thereby enabling them to move forward. This process, sometimes also referred to as alternative dispute resolution (ADR), is becoming increasingly popular in a wide range of settings, not least since Lord Justice Wolfe's report (1996) recommended its use in many legal disputes as an alternative to litigation.

It is important at the outset to say that social workers, advice workers and the various people-workers who seek to offer help, support, guidance and advice to people are not mediators in the strictest sense. Mediation as a discrete service is available to people who wish, or need to avail themselves of it, especially in cases of relationship breakdown, even though some areas of the country still do not have easy access to such services.

What is being suggested, however, is that mediation *skills* are much more generic, and are enormously important elements in your 'bag of skills' for dealing effectively with the conflict that is at the heart of a lot of people-work, no matter where you work.

This is not to assume that all conflict is necessarily bad. On the contrary, whenever we seek to change the way in which we, and others around us, behave, conflict is inevitable; all sorts of good changes and positive advances will involve a measure of conflict in order to effect positive change. The problems occur when the impact of conflict is negative; when people get stuck, refuse to budge, and take up positions that they will defend at all costs. Mediation skills are useful for defusing negative conflict, helping people to 'unhook' themselves from fixed positions and releasing a vision of what the future might be like if the conflict could be resolved creatively.

It would be wrong to assume that situations of conflict will only occur between people who use your services or whose relationships have seriously deteriorated. Some of the most debilitating conflicts for people-workers can be internal to their agency, where clashes of opinion or personality can make a team environment an unhappy, even toxic place to work. Managers often have to make difficult decisions about resource allocations, leading workers to feel sometimes that they have returned to the era of the 'deserving' and 'undeserving' poor.

Some conflicts are unresolvable, especially when you are trying to make finite resources stretch to meet seemingly infinite need, or where people stubbornly refuse to cooperate. Some people enjoy a good conflict or battle by having their day in court and handing over the ultimate decision to someone else, preferably a person in authority like a magistrate or judge, or an arbitrator. Some divorcing parents choose to have their residence and contact disputes decided by a court because one or other of the parents does not want to appear to their children to be giving up their parenting claim, and prefer to leave the decision for 'a wise judge' to make.

These examples are at the extreme end of the spectrum and in your everyday work you are more likely to come across less serious examples of conflict, where you could well make a considerable impact by a judicious use of mediation skills.

## Activity

Think of two or three examples of conflict you have experienced recently, where people have been in dispute. Ask yourself:

- What was the conflict about?
- What were the key issues involved?
- Why do you think those involved seemed unable to achieve an amicable outcome?

## ESSENTIAL SKILLS

### Active listening and clarifying

Unless you are able to listen really carefully, you will not be able to make much progress. Listening is not just about hearing and understanding what the disputants are saying to each other; it is also about listening for what each of them is *not* saying, the issues they are *not* raising. These are often at the heart of the conflict, because they indicate what each of the parties is frightened about. Conflicts often occur when people's interests are threatened or undermined in some way; they can get very defensive and aggressive at the prospect of losing out. It is important to note that such fears could be well founded, or completely irrational. Active listening will attempt to identify what the conflict is about; what the key issues are, and what is preventing them from reaching a workable solution.

Active listening is also a visual activity. You pick up 'non-verbal signals' from each of the disputants. How people look at each other; what hand gestures they make; how they sit; how they respond physically to what is being said or alleged – all reveal important information about what is going on inside each person and how they are feeling. At times, the non-verbal signals can contradict the words people use, and usually these will reveal what the person is *really* trying to communicate.

### Interpreting and clarifying

People in dispute do not always think clearly when they are under pressure; sentences sometimes come tumbling out in the heat of the moment that, on reflection, they would have preferred to have said differently. Sometimes words seem very inadequate tools to use to convey meaning fully. And when people are in the turbulence of an argument or dispute, there is no guarantee that each will hear clearly what the other is saying. Indeed, it is more than likely that on occasion they will seize on one aspect of what is being said to them, and ignore the rest. We can all 'get hold of the wrong end of the stick', and in disputes such sticks often seem to have more wrong ends than we would ever realise!

An important listening and communication skill, therefore, for someone who is 'in the middle' is to look for occasions when mishearing or miscommunication is taking place. This is an important role for you to play, checking out with those concerned whether that was really what they intended to say, or whether they had something else in mind. Sometimes the simple process of clarifying, and asking whether or not 'this or that' was what the person really intended, can play an important part in enabling disputants to listen to each other, rather than talk past each other. By undertaking this clarifying role, you may discover that people who have appeared unable to 'see the wood for the trees' begin to understand each other better. This is often the first step towards a resolution.

## Summarising

In the early stages of an argument, there may often be 'more heat than light', and from time to time it will be important for you to take some control of what is happening and to reflect back to each of the people how you see the story so far. This skill of summarising can serve a number of purposes:

- It reminds people that you are trying to help them to come to a solution.
- It can take the heat out of the situation, even if only briefly.
- It offers each of them a 'mirror' to see what impression they have been creating to an outsider.
- It provides an opportunity to 'listen back'. They can check whether your 'reflections' accurately represent what they intend to say or not. It does not matter too much whether you have got it completely right: if you have missed something, or got something wrong, they will be quick to point this out, and this will in itself aid further clarification.
- It provides an opportunity to decide on what the steps are to be in seeking a resolution.

## Mutualising, normalising and re-framing

Mutualising seeks to recognise common ground between the disputants. It can help them realise that, far from being poles apart, they may be closer to coming to a solution than they had realised. If you can demonstrate the common concerns and interests they share, it can often help people move forward. A classic example of this is when divorcing parents argue, sometimes bitterly, about what is best for their children. A mutualising statement would acknowledge that each of them as parents really loves the children and wants what is best for them.

Normalising can help people pull back from the brink. We often assume that the problems we encounter are so unique to us that they are in a different league from anyone else's. In one sense that is perfectly true: there is only one of us in the whole world and how we experience things will be unique to us. But the temptation when we are in a dispute is to ratchet up this claim to uniqueness, and to give the impression *that the problems and issues that we are raising are so different from anything else anyone else has ever experienced that it will be 'beyond the wit' of anyone to come up with a decent solution.* In other words, we place ourselves in what we believe is a safe place where only a total capitulation by the other person will suffice.

However, the difficulties people experience often have common themes or strands to them which can lead to a range of perfectly acceptable solutions. Sometimes people need reassuring that (at times) overwhelming feelings often go with the territory, but need not block a solution being found.

Re-framing Disputants naturally want to tell their own story from their own point of view. They will rehearse their version meticulously, to be fully heard and understood, and perhaps ensure that the other person is seen in a negative light. Re-framing involves suggesting, in non-judgemental ways, different perspectives. The previous example of two parents in dispute over their children would be a good example of this. If you can re-frame their stories so that each parent acknowledges their motivation to be a good parent, then this could lead to a solution-focused, mutual acknowledgement that each of them has the best interests of their children at heart.

Looking towards a 'win–win' outcome

Although there are sometimes conflicts and disputes where one person is clearly in the wrong, and the decision has to go against them, more often a solution is needed which both disputants can own. If one person 'wins hands down', the loser will feel demoralised, de-motivated and perhaps even humiliated. The best solutions, therefore, enable each person to walk away having fully expressed their concerns and points of view whilst having contributed to a mutually acceptable workable solution. This is clearly going to be important where people still need to work or live together. It is a skill, therefore, that anyone seeking to help resolve conflict needs to keep clearly in focus.

## Group exercise

With the help of your tutor or supervisor, discuss the scenarios identified in the Activity above, and explore ways in which mediation skills could help you work towards a resolution.

## FINAL THOUGHTS

No one pretends that you will find these skills easy to practise. At times, you will catch yourself taking sides. Your own experiences and feelings about conflict, and how you have emerged from disputes, will all influence how you behave when caught up in a mediating role with people in dispute. Sometimes to hold the middle ground is the hardest task of all, and requires perceptive supervision, but if you are to be an effective mediator, it is the only place to be.

## REFERENCES AND FURTHER READING

Brown, H. and Marriott, A. (2018) *ADR Principles and Practice*, 4th edition. London: Sweet & Maxwell.

Charlton, R. and Dewdney, M. (2014) *The Mediator's Handbook*, 3rd edition. Sydney: Lawbook Co.

Stewart, S. (1998) *Conflict Resolution: A Foundation Guide*. Winchester: Waterside Press.

Wolfe, Lord Justice (1996) *Access to Justice*, Final Report. London: The Lord Chancellor's Department.

**RELATED CONCEPTS** active listening; challenging; conflict management; empathy: dealing with upset service users; non-verbal communication

**ENGAGING WITH THE PCF** critical reflection and analysis; skills and interventions; professionalism; values and ethics

**ENGAGING WITH THE NMC CODE** promote professionalism and trust

---

### Service user snippet

Kevin (33), after attending a family mediation session:

'I hated the idea of both of us having to wash all our dirty linen in front of a complete stranger, but it seemed the only way to get things right for the kids. And in the end it wasn't that bad – they were very even-handed with us both, and I think we got it sorted OK.'

# MINDFULNESS

One of the hazards in people-work is the way in which our own thoughts, worries, anxieties and fears can get in the way when we are working with people who have their own distress to deal with. It is rather like having the volume turned up of any background music of our own lives so that we find it difficult to give our undivided attention to the other person. To put it starkly, we get in the way of the help we are seeking to give.

One of the important skills in communication, therefore, is the ability to turn down the volume of our own background noise, and to develop and practise a set of skills that enable this to happen. Learning how to relax mentally, seek an inner calm and stillness and consciously step aside from our own emotional or spiritual baggage, is an essential component to effective communication.

Each of us needs to discover what works best for us and how to prepare ourselves for the work we undertake with others. Music, going for a walk, using a labyrinth, various relaxation techniques, prayer and meditation – the list seems endless.

Increasing in popularity is the use of mindfulness, which has its roots in Buddhism but which now plays a significant role in cognitive behavioural therapy (CBT). Moffitt describes mindfulness as 'the ability to see clearly what needs to be done, what you are capable of doing, and how it relates to the larger truth of life' (2009, cited in Greer, 2016: 39). This is a definition that will resonate with any people-worker who has had to struggle with difficult and challenging scenarios, and relates immediately to the issues outlined above. By focusing on 'living in the moment' – a mindfulness phrase which challenges us to fine-tune our attention and thinking to what is immediately facing us – we can begin 'to move towards acknowledging what anxieties, fears and emotions are affecting how we are thinking and behaving. We can [then] take ourselves to a calm space from which we can make a wise decision' (Moffitt, 2009, cited in Greer, 2016: 30).

It is not appropriate in this short entry to explore mindfulness in great detail. What is important to emphasise is the responsibility we all have to ensure that we do not allow our own personal 'stuff' to intrude into our work with others. Mindfulness encourages us first of all to recognise what Greer (2016) calls our 'inner chatter and mental noise' and the ways in which it can seriously get in the way of the help, encouragement and support we seek to give to others. It reminds us that whether we like it or not, if we don't deal with this we will be communicating our own disquiet and unease to the other person who will assuredly pick it up from how we are behaving. Mindfulness also offers us an approach which seeks to deal with this crucial challenge to our effectiveness as communicators.

## Activity

Set aside 5 minutes each day when you consciously try to 'turn down your inner noise' and be still. Let your eyes and ears take in the sights and sounds around you. Be aware of your breathing and try to breathe slowly and deeply.

## Group exercise

With the help of your tutor or supervisor, undertake some research into mindfulness with some colleagues and find a book or a website (e.g. www.mindful.org) which appeals to you. Share your discoveries and discuss what might work best for you.

## FINAL THOUGHTS

Whether you choose mindfulness or another alternative approach is up to you, of course. Many would argue that in the major religious traditions the experience of meditation, prayer and being still has a similar powerful impact. But all of us have to be able to answer this basic question: How do we take active steps to ensure that we are dealing with our inner noise in such a way that it does not get in the way of the help we are seeking to offer?

## REFERENCES AND FURTHER READING

Brass, E. (2016) 'How mindfulness can benefit nursing practice', *Nursing Times*, 112 (18): 21–3.

Fleming, J.E. and Kocovski, N.L. (2013) *The Mindfulness and Acceptance Workbook*. Oakland, CA: New Harbinger.

Greer, J. (2016) *Resilience and Personal Effectiveness for Social Workers*. London: Sage. (See pp. 38–40; 106–11; 140–1.)

Moffitt, P. (2009) 'Mindfulness and compassion: tools for transforming suffering into joy', in P. Moffitt (ed.), *Dancing with Life*. Tiburon, CA: Dharma Wisdom, Life Balance Institute.

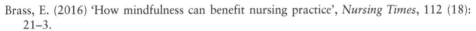

**RELATED CONCEPTS** active listening; empowerment, resilience and a strengths perspective; labyrinths; reflective practice

**ENGAGING WITH THE PCF** critical reflection and analysis; professionalism

**ENGAGING WITH THE NMC CODE** practise effectively; promote professionalism and trust

Service user snippet

Janine (21), newly qualified nurse:

'I was getting so stressed by the demands of the job – it was so busy and seeing people in distress was really getting to me – and then one of the more experienced nurses said "Why don't you have a go at this mindfulness lark? It's worth a try and works for me." She was right!'

# MOTIVATIONAL INTERVIEWING

Our attitude to change is often ambivalent. We would like to enjoy the benefits of a different lifestyle, but the journey we need to make can be daunting, even off-putting. If only fitness were instantaneously available *off the shelf* simply by paying the health club subscription. Hours needed on the treadmill somehow take the shine off the aspiration.

---

## Activity

Think about your own life and any changes you would like to achieve. How do you intend to go about it? What improvements do you hope to see? What holds you back or prevents you making these changes?

---

As you reflect on this Activity you may recognise that underneath the often complex factors affecting change, there is a simple equation: if motivation is outweighed by reluctance and resistance, change will not happen. It is not that you are a bad or sick person, or that there is something wrong with you: it's just that the balance needs significant shifting. If, however, the motivation is strong enough, then the chances of success are greatly enhanced.

Motivational interviewing helps people readjust the balance in the apparently conflicting or opposing influences which affect change. As a skilled intervention it is mainly associated with challenging addictive behaviours through the pioneering work of Miller and Rollnick (2012), but has wider implications for professional practice.

There is a further dimension which we all recognise: as Koprowska (2014: 22–3) observes, 'we do not like to be told what to do or how to behave'. There is a strong temptation among professionals to adopt the role of expert and tell people what to do, and this is so often counter-productive. Motivational interviewing seeks to challenge such an approach.

An important first step in understanding motivational change is the value base of the person seeking to give help and how this influences their attitude to the person in need. In their work with 'problem drinkers', Miller and Rollnick (2012) challenged the 'disease' or 'deficient personality' approaches, and instead sharpened up a particular counselling approach that has now become known as motivational interviewing (MI). With its roots in Carl Rogers's client-centred approach (1951), MI stresses the importance first of all of an empathic stance. You need fully to understand where the other person 'is coming from' – their hopes and fears that underlie their wish to change but also fuel their resistance and reluctance. You should not be surprised when people express deep ambivalence to change; on the contrary (as we all know from our own experience) it is pretty normal. Deep empathy encapsulates the value base of the listener and affirms the value of the person seeking to change.

In her summary of the next steps in MI, Trevithick (2012: 333–6) highlights three key themes. The first is to encourage the person seeking change to put into words how they see the tension between what they want to happen and what is holding them back, and then to present the argument for change. This can be challenging and painful, and the 'helper' needs to be comfortable in being directive at this point. MI suggests that it is this ability to put into their own words this 'discrepancy' that is the key to making progress.

Second, the helper will avoid telling people what to do or trying to persuade them to achieve various outcomes, but will focus instead on the energy inherent in the resistance to change. In sporting terms, a wrestler will seek to gain advantage from an opponent's resistance by changing direction and allowing the opponent's body weight to work in moving them in a different direction. In MI the emphasis is on exploring resistance and to help the person find their own solutions and outcomes. How can they rechannel all the energy currently reinforcing their resistance and redirect it towards a different outcome?

Third, this approach reflects what MI calls 'self-efficacy' or the person's self-belief in their ability to make change and to succeed. It echoes the emphasis in much contemporary people-work upon a strengths perspective, empowerment and resilience. At its root therefore, MI challenges all people-workers to examine their approach to resistance. Instead of adopting a blaming or negative stereotyping approach, resistance is almost welcomed as normal, something to be expected, and to be worked with in a positive way so that the power balance can be shifted in another direction.

## Group exercise

With the help of your tutor or supervisor, explore various scenarios where MI would be helpful (e.g. dealing with loss; experiencing rejection; struggling to deal with addiction). In small groups, discuss how you would approach each scenario.

## FINAL THOUGHTS

There is one further dimension to this discussion that is less prominent in the literature. Empathy is an important way of valuing and strengthening the other person's self-belief. Often low self-esteem negates successful motivation. There are, however, spiritual and sometimes religious dimensions to this, especially when one of the 'blocks' involves a feeling of sinfulness and unredeemable wrongdoing. In such situations, a seeking-out and accepting of forgiveness can lead to a liberating release of energy that boosts motivation and the journey towards change (Holloway and Moss, 2010: 135–6). Gentle challenges to a person's sense of unworthiness therefore is another crucial aspect of the empathic role of MI.

## REFERENCES AND FURTHER READING

Holloway, M. and Moss, B. (2010) *Spirituality and Social Work*. Basingstoke: Palgrave Macmillan.
Koprowska, J. (2014) *Communication and Interpersonal Skills in Social Work*, 4th edition. Exeter: Learning Matters.
Miller, W.R. and Rollnick, S. (2012) *Motivational Interviewing: Helping People Change*, 3rd edition. London: Guilford Press.
Rogers, C.R. (1951) *Client-Centred Therapy*. London: Constable.
Trevithick, P. (2012) *Social Work Skills and Knowledge: A Practice Handbook*, 3rd edition. Maidenhead: Open University Press.

**RELATED CONCEPTS** empathy; empowerment, resilience and a strengths perspective; religion; spirituality

**ENGAGING WITH THE PCF** professional leadership; skills and interventions; values and ethics

**ENGAGING WITH THE NMC CODE** promote professionalism and trust

### Service user snippet

Sean (34), youth worker:

'I can't tell you how stuck I was – didn't know which way to turn – it was getting me down big time ... but then someone at work suggested I give this motivational interviewing lark a try ... and what a difference – I feel like a new man and at last I know where I am going.'

# NON-VERBAL COMMUNICATION

It is often said that a picture is worth a thousand words. By this is meant that a picture can convey in breadth and depth a far wider and more complex set of meanings in its constricted space on the canvas than would be possible by just using words alone. This is not meant to diminish the power of words; rather, it paints for us a wider context in which communication takes place.

If, for a moment, we regard our physical body as a picture that we are presenting to the people with whom we work, then a similar point can be made. What we communicate to that person is more than the actual words we use: it is the whole bundle of messages, signals and symbols that our physical presence conveys. Whatever words a police officer or traffic warden may use when challenging us with a misdemeanour, it will be the symbol of their uniform that makes the greatest impact upon us. This conveys the very clear message: *mess with me at your peril*.

In her important discussion of non-verbal communication, Trevithick (2012: 166ff) refers to a study by Mehrabian (1972), who estimated that in a typical encounter involving two people, 'the overall communication is made up of body language (55 per cent); paralanguage (non-verbal aspects of speech) 38 per cent and the verbal 7 per cent'. This has profound implications for anyone involved in people-work. It is not saying that the words we use are unimportant – far from it. But it is suggesting that our words are only some of the paints we use to produce the picture of our interaction with someone, and that non-verbal communication skills are likely to be far more dominant, and have a far greater impact overall.

Some examples will help to illustrate the point:

- As a nurse you are sitting with someone who has recently been bereaved. There is nothing you can say to alleviate their distress, but you sit quietly and allow them to talk or cry, or to be silent. When you leave, you are surprised to hear them say to you how much they have appreciated your visit and how helpful it has been.
- A social worker goes to court to present a report on a young person, turning up dressed in a sloppy pullover and jeans, and is asked by the magistrates to leave the court.
- A female worker in a men's bail hostel turns up to help run a group-work session wearing a low-cut FCUK top and a mini skirt, and is asked by the manager to go home and come back dressed more appropriately.
- A community worker arrives to visit a family with massive debt problems and a range of other difficulties, dressed in a sharp expensive suit and gold cufflinks and carrying an expensive leather briefcase, and is surprised by the cold reception he receives.

## Activity

Discuss the four scenarios outlined above. What do you think are the key issues with each of them in terms of non-verbal communication? Do you agree with the decisions taken in the second and third scenarios?

These scenarios illustrate the point that, in each case, the person involved was communicating a very powerful message about themselves non-verbally, which was picked up and responded to. It is important to note that these examples – and indeed this whole discussion – are focusing only on non-verbal communication in a professional or work-based setting, and the roles that we fulfil.

Non-verbal communication through how we dress or behave is also an issue in our personal and social lives, but there are different issues involved there which are not quite so relevant to this discussion. Nevertheless, it has to be said that, whether in a professional or personal context, the way a person dresses should never be regarded as an invitation to any unacceptable or threatening behaviour.

Before going into more detail, it is important to stress that we do have control over our non-verbal communication, and that it can rightly be regarded as a communication skill. How we dress says something very important to the people with whom we come into contact. The various settings you become involved in have a significant impact upon how you dress and present yourselves. You need to give some thought to this. To turn up in a formal setting, such as court, shabbily dressed is not only going to be regarded as disrespectful to the court, it also runs the risk of doing a major disservice to the person you are seeking to represent or support. A 'take it or leave it' or 'this is not something to get worked up about' approach, conveyed by the casual attire, is not the message the court expects you to give.

It is important to recognise the *context* of your work with people, and the non-verbal messages that can be conveyed. For example, you are conveying non-verbal messages in all of the following ways:

- whether you are punctual for your appointments, and keep to the time allotted for your visit or interview;
- how you dress and the appearance you present to people;
- how you arrange the room if you are meeting people at the office;
- whether you offer a symbolic touch to people, such as a handshake;
- how you manage the space or distance between yourself and the other person;
- whether you offer refreshments to people;
- how you sit; your posture, and how you move; whether or not you fidget;
- whether or not you smile; your facial expressions and gestures;
- how you bring the meeting to a close and take your leave.

There are other non-verbal aspects of communication that can be important from time to time. For example:

- When you visit a person in their own home, wait to be shown where they would like you to sit; allow a pause for them to clear away any clutter.
- If there is a dog in the house and you are fearful of it, wait at the door until it is taken into another room.
- If the television is on and it is difficult to hear what is being said and you feel awkward about asking for it to be turned down, try moving your face closer to the person who is speaking, and glance at the TV – maybe point at the TV, and make a minimising gesture with your hand to invite it to be turned down or off. (Of course, if you feel able to ask them directly to turn it down or off, then this can be so much easier!)
- Make a point of switching your mobile phone onto silent or vibrate mode in front of the other person. This tells them that you are giving them undivided time, but also makes it clear that you can make a call if you need help or assistance.
- If you have any uncertainty about the person you are interviewing, ensure that you have an easy exit route by placing yourself near to the door.

So far, we have concentrated on the skills that you need to develop across a wide range of non-verbal communication, and we have suggested that careful attention to these will help to ensure a much more successful outcome to your meetings or interviews. Certainly, if there is congruence between the non-verbal and verbal content of your interview, you will have been pretty effective in the task you have had to complete. By contrast, if the non-verbal signs and signals have contradicted what you have said, the 'non-verbals' will win 'hands down'.

Non-verbal communication also works in the other direction, of course. You can tell a lot about the other person by 'reading the signs' accurately: how a person is dressed and how they present themselves; what their living conditions are like; how they greet you; how they hold themselves physically; how they respond to you. All these are signs and clues about how the other person is feeling, which can help you in your communication and assessment.

## NON-VERBAL SKILLS FOR HANDLING AGGRESSION

One particularly difficult area where non-verbal communication is of central importance is in dealing with aggression. If someone becomes agitated, and starts jabbing a finger at you or waving a clenched fist, if they begin to raise their voice and start talking more quickly, or suddenly get up from their seat, you don't need much insight to realise that aggression is mounting, and that you may be at risk. Accident and emergency departments at busy weekends often witness violent behaviour against staff, and attacks against people-workers are becoming increasingly common. This is therefore an important issue for you to explore.

Your first priority must be for your own safety, and you may need to activate the panic button (if you are in the office context) or simply leave the room to seek help and escape the threat of violence.

There are, however, a number of non-verbal responses that you can use which may help to defuse the situation, even though quite understandably you will feel nervous or afraid. A lot may depend, of course, on the gender mix of the interview: sometimes women can more easily defuse a situation when a man begins to show anger and aggression, but whatever the situation there are some guidelines that will prove helpful. These include:

- Try to remain calm and breathe deeply.
- Stand up if the other person stands up, but avoid adopting a confrontational posture.
- Ask the person by name to sit down; tell them that their behaviour makes it difficult for you to concentrate, and that you want to discuss what is bothering them.
- Speak and move a little more slowly than usual to help the other person slow down.
- Keep at a reasonable distance from the other person – out of arm's reach, if possible.
- Do not attempt to touch the other person; keep your own hands and arms relaxed.
- Keep looking straight at the other person without staring, or smiling (this can sometimes be interpreted as mocking).
- Keep as still, relaxed and calm as possible.
- If you feel comfortable, sit down and invite the other person to sit so that you can resume your discussion.
- When things calm down a bit, ask if they would like a few minutes to collect their thoughts before you resume your discussion; maybe they would like a drink (be careful though – you do not want hot cups of tea being thrown at you later on).

These are a few suggestions on how best to cope, and how to use non-verbal communication skills to defuse an aggressive situation. We repeat our initial advice, however: if you feel threatened and at risk, your first responsibility is to remove yourself from the situation as quickly as possible.

## Group exercise

With the help of your tutor or supervisor, discuss as a group how you would handle an aggressive situation. Check your agency or hospital guidelines, procedures and lone-worker policies as part of its health and safety policy. Draw up your own guidelines for best practice.

## FURTHER THOUGHTS

For people without speech, those who are deaf or hearing impaired, and those with specific communication difficulties, non-verbal communication is their main means of relating to other people. Many of the issues already raised in this discussion still remain relevant, but the principal means of communication will be different. British

Sign Language (BSL), for example, is a language in its own right, celebrated and used by the deaf community. It is a beautiful, 'liquid' flowing form of communication using fingers, hands and facial gestures. For deafblind people, the language of BSL is communicated through touch. Makaton is an artificial system for basic communication that has been devised to help people without speech, or with limited verbal capacity, to communicate with others.

The advent of electronic and computer technology has enabled many people without speech to become far more fluent in their communication skills. Many disabled people can now use the computer to communicate, even if they have limited or no manual dexterity. By using pointers that they can operate by mouth or as an attachment to their foreheads, they are able to develop communication skills which have enhanced their quality of life.

## REFERENCES AND FURTHER READING

Koprowska, J. (2014) *Communication and Interpersonal Skills in Social Work*, 4th edition. Exeter: Learning Matters.

Mehrabian, A. (1972) *Nonverbal Communication*. Chicago, IL: Aldine.

Trevithick, P. (2012) *Social Work Skills: A Practice Handbook*, 3rd edition. Maidenhead: Open University Press.

Williams, P. (2009) *Social Work with People with Learning Difficulties*, 2nd edition. Exeter: Learning Matters.

Woodcock Ross, J. (2016) *Specialist Communication Skills for Social Workers: Developing Professional Capability*, 2nd edition. Basingstoke: Palgrave Macmillan.

**RELATED CONCEPTS** barrier gestures; conflict management; empathy: dealing with upset service users; establishing a professional relationship; reflective practice

**ENGAGING WITH THE PCF** context and organisations; critical reflection and analysis; skills and interventions; professionalism

**ENGAGING WITH THE NMC CODE** practise effectively; promote professionalism and trust

### Service user snippet

Sonia (19), prison interview:

'I could tell straightaway he wasn't really interested in what I had to say … he just sat there in his nice suit and posh briefcase … and kept staring out of the window when I stopped talking … I could of [sic] smacked him.'

# OVERCOMING FEARS AND ANXIETIES

## PROFESSOR LIZ BOATH

Communication can be a major source of anxiety and unless it is recognised and dealt with your ability to communicate effectively will be seriously undermined. One example of this is *glossophobia*, or the fear of public speaking. This is extremely common and intense and is perhaps the single most common fear that people express. So if you suffer from this, take comfort from the knowledge that you are not alone.

Fear of public speaking not only affects you physiologically – a dry mouth, increased blood pressure, blushing, sweating, trembling, racing heart and irregular breathing – but also emotionally, as you fear humiliation and looking foolish. Women also report higher rates of social anxiety than men (Furmark, 2002). In addition, social anxiety prevents people from applying for, taking or doing the job they are really good at doing.

However, the good news is that fears and anxieties can be overcome. It is therefore essential that a book on communication skills includes ideas on how to deal with fears and anxieties around communication. So, whether you have full-blown social anxiety or just get a little anxious, this tried and tested method can help you.

It is important if your anxiety levels are extremely high, or you feel that you need support with your anxiety, that you contact your GP, who can refer you for help or support. However, the strategies outlined below may help.

## EMOTIONAL FREEDOM TECHNIQUES (EFT/TAPPING)

Emotional freedom techniques (EFT), also known as 'tapping', is a new and evolving psychological intervention that can help with social anxiety (Stewart et al, 2013). It is a very gentle therapy that is simple to learn and easy to use. You gently tap with your fingertips on acupressure points on your head, torso and hands and relate this to the voicing of specific statements (Craig, 2011). These are a range of studies using EFT focusing on social anxiety and public speaking anxiety (e.g. Jones et al., 2011; Boath et al., 2012). It has also been used to reduce presentation anxiety with social work students (Boath et al., 2017). So, why not take 15 minutes to test out tapping for yourself using the following example?

# Activity

The images below show you the tapping points. Please have a go at tapping gently 5–7 times on each point.

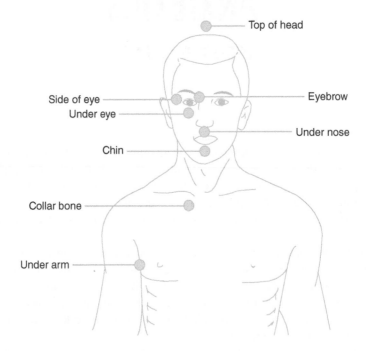

**Figure 7** Tapping points

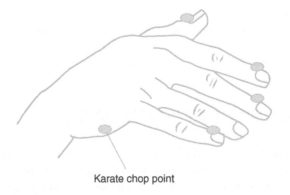

Karate chop point

**Figure 8** Hand tapping points

Now, focus on your feelings:

1    First of all, decide the best way to describe how you are feeling *right now*. Try to be as specific as you can. Ask yourself the following questions, and write down the answers:

i    *What* emotion am I feeling? (e.g. anxiety, fear, worry, panic, etc.)

ii   *Where* do I feel it? (e.g. chest, shoulders, throat, stomach, etc.)

iii  *What* does it feel like? (e.g. a lump in your throat; a tingling in your arms; a churning in your stomach)

iv   Do any *shapes*, *colours*, *textures*, *names*, *words*, etc. come to mind when I think about my feeling? (e.g. red, churning anxiety)

v    What is the *intensity* of my feeling? Rate this on a scale of 0–10, with 0 being no intensity and 10 being the worst ever (e.g. level 8).

Now, put all these together to make your *set-up statement*. For example:

'Even though I am feeling anxious, in my chest, a red, churning anxiety at a level of 8, that's just the way it is for now.'

2    While continuously tapping on the outside of your hand (karate-chop point), say your set-up statement three times.

3    Gently tap about 5–7 times on each of the *tapping points*. Do this in the order shown on the diagram above. Restate your issue (this is called the *reminder phrase*) on each tapping point.

For example:

'Anxiety in my chest.'

'This red, churning, anxiety.'

'Anxiety at a level of 8.'

'All this anxiety in my chest.'

'All this anxiety I'm feeling.'

'This anxiety.'

4    Take a deep breath and relax!

5    Focus on what you are feeling now and make any changes, for example, it might have changed to a 'smaller pink ball of anxiety in my throat at a level of 6'. It is important to tap on what you are experiencing now, so if the colour, feeling or emotion changes, change the words you use.

6    Repeat the tapping process in step 3 and revise the phrase you use accordingly.

7    Write down how anxious you feel right now. Has the level of anxiety gone down? Keep tapping and see if it does, or if you can reduce it further.

*Note*: If you need to seek further help with EFT, it is essential that you work with a qualified and accredited practitioner. You can find a list of practitioners at https://eftinternational.org/discover-eft-tapping/find-eft-practitioners/ (accessed 23/10/19). For a free EFT handbook, see Web resources below.

## Group exercise

With the help of your tutor or supervisor, why not set up a group and invite your colleagues to explore 'tapping' and then share what hints and tips work best for them?

## FINAL THOUGHT

You won't know if you don't try!

## REFERENCES AND FURTHER READING

Boath, E., Good, R., Tsaroucha, A., Stewart, T., Pitch, S. and Boughey, A.J. (2017) 'Tapping your way to success: using emotional freedom techniques (EFT) to reduce anxiety and improve communication skills in social work students', *Social Work Education*, 36 (6): 715–30.

Boath, E.H., Stewart, A. and Carryer, A. (2012) 'Tapping for PEAS: emotional freedom technique (EFT) in reducing presentation expression anxiety syndrome (PEAS) in university students', *Innovative Practice in Higher Education*, 1 (2): 1–12. Available at www.staffs. ac.uk/ipihe (accessed 23/02/17).

Boath, E.H., Stewart, A. and Carryer, A. (2013) 'Tapping for success: emotional freedom techniques (EFT) for enhancing academic performance in university students', *Innovative Practice in Higher Education*, 1 (3). Available at www.staffs.ac.uk/ipihe (accessed 23/02/17).

Craig, G. (2011) *The EFT Manual*, 2nd edition. Fulton, CA: Energy Psychology Press.

Furmark, T. (2002) 'Social phobia: overview of community surveys', *Acta Psychiatrica Scandinavica*, 105 (2): 84–93.

Jones, S., Thornton, J. and Andrews, H. (2011) 'Efficacy of emotional freedom techniques (EFT) in reducing public speaking anxiety: a randomized controlled trial', *Energy Psychology: Theory, Research, Treatment*, 3 (1).

Stewart, A., Boath, E.H., Carryer, A., Walton, I. and Hill, L. (2013) 'Can emotional freedom techniques (EFT) be effective in the treatment of emotional conditions? Results of a service evaluation in Sandwell', *Psychological Therapies in Primary Care*, 2 (1): 71–84.

### Web resources

EFT, free Tapping Handbook: https://eftinternational.org/discover-eft-tapping/free-eft-manual/ (accessed 15/10/19)

EFT, Discover the latest research: https://eftinternational.org/discover-eft-tapping/eft-science-research/ (accessed 15/10/19)

**RELATED CONCEPTS** empowerment, resilience and a strengths perspective; talks and presentations

**ENGAGING WITH THE PCF** critical reflection and analysis

**ENGAGING WITH THE NMC CODE** practise effectively; promote professionalism and trust

## Service user snippet

Christian (21), student:

'I dreaded having to give a presentation as part of my course, and to be honest when I heard of this tapping malarky I thought it was daft. But it worked – it really did! AND I got a decent mark.'

# PROFESSIONAL CAPABILITIES FRAMEWORK (PCF)

Sometimes we cannot see the wood for the trees. We become so caught up with the minutiae of everyday practice that we lose sight of the overall picture, something which Thompson (2012) calls 'helicopter vision'. We need sometimes to regain sight of the horizons and boundaries of our work. This is why the Professional Capabilities Framework (PCF), developed originally for social workers in England in 2012 by The College of Social Work (TCSW), was devised. Since the demise of TCSW, the PCF has been taken over by the British Association of Social Workers (BASW) and following extensive consultation a refreshed PCF was developed.

The PCF is a graphic pictorial overview of the complexity and richness of professional practice, from a social work point of view – though other professionals can also derive benefit from exploring it. Wherever you are in your social work career – student, newly qualified social worker, experienced social worker or manager – you will be located somewhere on the PCF and can gain an overview of the knowledge, skills and values that are appropriate to your role and status within the organisation. The nine domains are intended to convey the richness and complexity of professional practice but they are not watertight compartments – they all blend together, each enhancing the rest (see Figure 9). As Woodcock Ross observes:

> The PCF brings a new developmental approach to assessment, with social workers' increasing *capacity* or *potential* to learn and adapt to increasingly complex situations and demands being a distinguishing feature. (Woodcock Ross, 2016: 29, citing Higgins and Goodyer, 2014; original emphasis)

If you go onto the BASW website (www.basw.co.uk) you will find the diagram of the PCF that allows you to locate your professional position (e.g. social worker, student, etc.). It is important to appreciate the significance of the nine domains, each one of which highlights an important aspect of the social worker's role and task. This refreshed PCF clusters the 9 domains into three super domains: Purpose, Practice and Impact. *Purpose* highlights why social workers do what they do; *Practice* holds together the skills, knowledge, interventions and critical abilities. From the communication perspective two things deserve mention: first, when you explore this super domain you will find communication skills and the level of complexity that is appropriate to your role level; and second, there are communication skills implications for each and every domain which need to be taken seriously. *Impact* shows how social workers can make a difference, and effect change through practice and professional leadership.

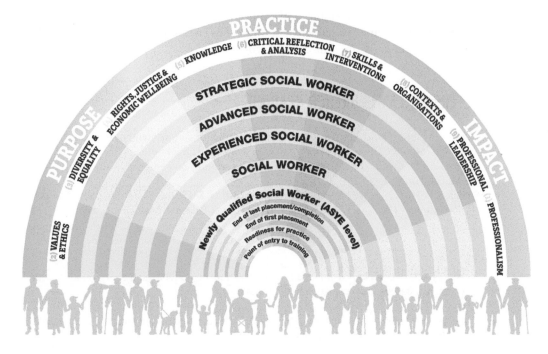

**Figure 9**   Professional Capabilities Framework (PCF) for social workers

*Source*: © British Association of Social Workers, 2018. Published with kind permission of BASW – www.basw.co.uk.

## Activity

Access the PCF via the BASW website (www.basw.co.uk). Locate your role level and carefully explore each domain, exploring the implications for your professional development. Where do you feel your strengths lie? What areas would benefit from further training? How will you negotiate this with your manager/supervisor/practice educator?

## Group exercise

With the help of your tutor or supervisor, compare the PCF with the NMC Code, described in the Introduction. What are the similarities or common themes? Compare and contrast these two approaches. What impresses you about each one?

## FINAL THOUGHTS

The underlying themes for the PCF, which are equally relevant to any people-work professional, reflect the levels of confidence you bring to your work, the ways in which you handle ambiguity and complexity in your professional practice, your developing skills in autonomous decision making and dealing with risk, and the ways in which your leadership and authority is nurtured and developed. In other words, the PCF is an invaluable tool designed to encourage you to achieve the highest possible standards in your chosen profession.

## REFERENCES AND FURTHER READING

Higgins, M. and Goodyer, A. (2014) 'The contradictions of contemporary social work: an ironic response', *British Journal of Social Work*, 45 (2): 747–60.

Thompson, N. (2012) *The People Solutions Sourcebook*, 2nd edition. Basingstoke: Palgrave Macmillan.

Woodcock Ross, J. (2016) *Specialist Communication Skills for Social Workers: Developing Professional Capability*, 2nd edition. Basingstoke: Palgrave Macmillan.

**RELATED CONCEPTS** anti-discriminatory practice; establishing a professional relationship; reflective practice; values and ethics

*Footnote for nurses*: You may wish to look again at the NMC Standards of Proficiency for Registered Nurses on the NMC website.

# REFLECTIVE PRACTICE

In the Introduction, you will have noted the emphasis that was laid upon reflective practice and its importance to your professional development. Two visual metaphorical images will help to make this point: reflective practice serves as a *mirror* and as a *video replay* in order to improve your professional practice.

## THE MIRROR

This image emphasises the importance of self-awareness in people-work. You need to know yourself well enough to ensure that the particular facets of your life enhance rather than detract from your effectiveness as a worker. Some of these facets are obvious: your age, race, gender, how you dress, the style of language you use and your accent; these all go to make up the 'real you', and they will have an impact upon the people you work with. You always hope that such facets will not get in the way of the work you do, but sometimes they will, and you need to be aware of this.

---

### Activity

Using this metaphorical image, look at yourself in the 'mirror' and list the characteristics you observe. Have there been occasions when these have been a distinct advantage in your people-work? Have there been occasions when they have got in the way? Are you able to understand why?

---

Less obvious are other facets of your personality that emerge during your meetings with people, and which perhaps are drawn out of you by the other person. Your likes and dislikes, your assumptions, fears and prejudices are good examples of this. Unfortunately, if you are not aware of these, they are likely to seep out and affect your relationships with people, either through what you say, or perhaps more likely through your non-verbal communication. An honest appraisal of your true self, 'warts and all', through this mirror of reflective practice, therefore, will help you to see where you need to be doubly careful in your dealings with others to ensure that you deliver best practice.

## VIDEO REPLAY

In your training, you may well have had the opportunity to video a simulated role-play interview to see yourself at work. There may be training opportunities in your present agency to do this. Less likely, because it is complicated by issues around confidentiality and data protection, is the opportunity to video yourself in a live interview, although in some family therapy settings this is often a useful tool.

When we talk here about video replay as a feature of reflective practice, however, we are using the term metaphorically. We are suggesting that in supervision and in training events, as well as in your own personal reflection on your practice, you 're-live' the interview and think about the following issues:

- What went well?
- What might you have done differently?
- What opportunities did you seize and which did you perhaps miss?
- What feelings were stirred up in you and the other person by the content of the interview, and how did you both handle these?
- How clear were your aims and objectives for the interview? Did you feel you achieved these? If so, how? If not, what got in the way?
- What issues for further reflection were brought up for you in this interview?

Note that the first question is about what went well. It is too easy to focus on the things you feel you did not do so well, but very rarely is an interview a complete disaster. Reflective practice is just as much about confirming the skills you do have and the confidence you can show as it is about exploring ways of improving your practice. Unfortunately, many people-workers, especially early on in their careers, need a lot of convincing that they can do the job well. Perhaps it is better than being over-confident, but an honest assessment of what you can do well is an important aspect of being a reflective practitioner.

The concept of being and becoming a reflective practitioner owes much to the seminal work of Schön (1983, 1987). He used the graphic image of the 'swampy lowlands' to describe the messy business of people-work with all its problems and complications. This he contrasted with the high ground of theory and research where problems are often much more easily resolved. The skill of being a reflective practitioner, however, is to make as full use as possible of relevant theoretical perspectives and research findings in order to help those in the swampy lowlands to work towards a creative and workable set of solutions to their difficulties.

Another seminal writer was Kolb (1984), who produced a diagrammatic model about adult learning that can very usefully also be applied to reflective practice (see Figure 10).

His box diagram has four components to it, with each leading to the next. As Thompson (2009: 74–5) explains, these four main aspects are:

1   *Concrete* day-to-day *experience* forms the first step in a chain of learning.

2   *Reflective observation* of our experience helps us begin to draw out the learning points.

3   *Abstract conceptualisation* involves forming links between the new experience and previous learning and experience. These links build up a 'mini theory' or conceptual framework.

4   In *active experimentation*, a cycle of learning is completed when new ideas are tried out in practice.

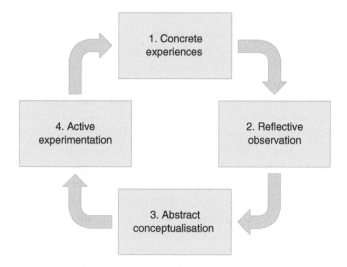

**Figure 10**   Kolb's cycle of learning (1984)

*Source*: Kolb, David A., Experiential Learning: Experience as the Source of Learning and Development, 2nd Edition © 2015. Reprinted by permission of Pearson Education, Inc., New York, New York.

---

## Group exercise

With the help of your tutor or supervisor, work in pairs with each choosing an example from your own practice to see how Kolb's cycle of learning might help you reflect upon, understand and improve your practice. Share your insights with the rest of the group.

---

## REFLECTIVE OR REFLEXIVE?

Much of the discussion so far has focused on what Schön (1983, 1987) called 'reflection-on-action', but there is a further dimension which he refers to as 'reflection-*in*-action'. This is a much more immediate Activity: it involves the 'here and now' of a practice situation where you have to 'think on your feet' and sometimes take immediate decisions. It may feel, on such occasions, that your values, your communication skills and your theoretical understanding all go into overdrive. Not only that, but the immediate impact you, as a worker, are having upon the person you are working with also comes strongly into play as you seek to take all of this into account. Some writers (such as Rolfe et al., 2011) argue that reflection-in-action should be regarded as *reflexive* practice, and you will often come across this term in the communication skills literature.

## ANOTHER METAPHOR: THE CREATIVE FOOTBALLER

For this reason, it is useful to introduce a third metaphorical image to help you understand this dimension of reflective practice: the creative football player. Here is the immediacy or reflection-in-action: the ball is at your feet; you need to be aware of everything and everyone who is around you; you need to have the vision to see where the game is going, and where to pass the ball to greatest effect. What happens next depends upon the decisions you take, and how other people react to you. After the match, you may well watch the video replay and realise that with the wisdom of hindsight you could have acted differently, but in the heat of the moment you did your best to use all your skills and previous knowledge to best effect.

Thompson and Thompson (2008: 24–6) capture the importance of this when they discuss openness as a core theme in reflective practice. They argue for openness of knowledge that is not fixed, dogmatic and closed but open to challenge and scrutiny and to the enrichment of further development; open-mindedness as a core approach to our practice, and openness to learning whereby we not only learn from our mistakes but can celebrate what we know we do well.

This approach takes us into the importance of critical reflection, whereby we bring a creative questioning approach to what we do and why we do it, and importantly what are some of the wider societal perspectives that impact upon our effectiveness. Reflective practice is not just about our individual performance: it is also about how we operate in a context where discrimination and oppression are powerful influences; where managerialism and scarce resources can seriously limit what we are able to do, and where (as Thompson, 2015: 184–93 warns) powerful structures can sometimes reinforce existing patterns of inequality and disadvantage.

These stark warnings are not meant to discourage you. Far from it; they are intended to help you locate your professional practice in the messy, turbulent and sometimes hostile context of contemporary society, and to offer you a creative way forward.

It is now essential for social workers to demonstrate critical reflective skills when seeking to re-register with the Health and Care Professions Council (HCPC). You need to demonstrate how your ongoing CPD activities have made an impact upon your practice. You will find the e-portfolio resources provided by TCSW invaluable as a reflective journal for developing and recording your reflective practice skills.

## FINAL THOUGHTS

There is a temptation in all people-work, especially when the sheer volume of work puts you under severe pressure, just to 'get on with it', to become almost mechanistic in your approach. The next person or patient, just like all those who have gone before, is 'just another case', and you deal with them as best you can before moving quickly on to the next. Perhaps what you need, as part of your commitment to best practice, is the mirror in which you creatively imagine that the next person you see is you, or one of your children, or one of your relatives. For many workers, that simple but powerful reminder is enough to rekindle their commitment to best practice, and to ensure that on a regular basis they reflect carefully on what they are doing and how they are doing it, so that everyone receives the best possible standard of help, care and support. As Thompson (2015: 264) explains, 'A reflective practitioner is a worker who is able to use experience, knowledge and theoretical perspectives to guide and inform practice'.

## REFERENCES AND FURTHER READING

Knott, C. and Scragg, T. (2016) *Reflective Practice in Social Work*, 4th edition. Exeter: Learning Matters.
Kolb, D.A. (1984) *Experiential Learning: Experience as the Source of Learning and Development*. London: Prentice Hall.
Rolfe, G., Freshwater, D. and Jasper, M. (2011) *Critical Reflection in Practice: Generating Knowledge for Care*, 2nd edition. Basingstoke: Palgrave Macmillan.
Schön, D. (1983) *The Reflective Practitioner*. New York: Basic Books.
Schön, D. (1987) *Educating the Reflective Practitioners*. San Francisco, CA: Jossey-Bass.
Thompson, N. (2009) *People Skills*, 3rd edition. Basingstoke: Palgrave Macmillan
Thompson, N. (2015) *People Skills*, 4th edition. Basingstoke: Palgrave Macmillan.
Thompson, S. and Thompson, N. (2008) *The Critically Reflective Practitioner*. Basingstoke: Palgrave Macmillan.
Woodcock Ross, J. (2016) *Specialist Communication Skills for Social Workers: Developing Professional Capability*, 2nd edition. Basingstoke: Palgrave Macmillan.

Web resource

British Association of Social Workers, Professional Capabilities Framework – www.basw.co.uk/professional-development/professional-capabilities-framework-pcf (accessed 15/10/19).

**RELATED CONCEPTS** anti-discriminatory practice; establishing a professional relationship; feedback: giving and receiving; labyrinth; Professional Capabilities Framework; supervision

**ENGAGING WITH THE PCF** critical reflection and analysis; values and ethics

**ENGAGING WITH THE NMC CODE** practise effectively; promote professionalism and trust

## Service user snippet

Gary (19), social work student:

'When I started I wondered what all the fuss was about – surely you just got on with it and did your best – but then I got a massive wake-up call on placement when one of my cases went pear-shaped and it was only when my supervisor sat me down and made me think through what had happened and how my values and attitudes had impacted on my poor practice that I saw why reflective practice had been drummed into us from day one.'

# RELIGION

You may feel surprised, shocked even, to find an entry on religion in a book devoted to communication skills. You may feel that religion is very much a private and personal matter, and that it does not have any bearing upon your work.

This view, however, needs to be challenged, and you need to develop the communication skills necessary to feel comfortable about exploring religious issues, when appropriate, with people who come to you for help and support. It is also important to acknowledge that one of the motivating factors drawing some people into a people-work career is often their religious faith. Social work has its origins in religious philanthropy, and medical and nursing care also has strong roots within religious traditions.

This is not to suggest that you must become a religious expert; but it is saying that the days when anything to do with religion was regarded as being 'off the radar' have long gone. In the 2011 UK census, for example, over 33 million people revealed that they would call themselves Christian and 2.7 million Muslim. Religion is generally regarded as a set of beliefs which are focused upon a divine power or being, and which binds a group of believers together into a shared community relationship. It also provides a particular interpretation of how the world is to be seen and understood. Believers will share this common world view, and often seek to persuade others of its validity. Alongside what are often referred to as 'major' religious faiths such as Christianity and Islam, for example, there is a plethora of other religious faiths and traditions which attract people's allegiance worldwide. The picture is bewilderingly complex, and it is no wonder perhaps that many people-workers do not know how to 'get started' when dealing with such matters.

## Activity

To help you engage with this issue, it is important to 'locate' yourself and to say where you stand on the issue of religion. For example: Are you yourself, or members of your family, religious? Can you say why this is important to you? If you are not, can you say why this is not important for you?

If religion is not important to you, you need to think about why some people feel differently. For instance:

- Some will say that their faith is central to their way of life, and provides them with a way of looking at, and understanding, the world and their place in it – in other words, it gives them their world view.

- In our multi-faith society, many people belong to a faith community where they receive, and give, support to each other in good times and bad. Their religion also embraces and celebrates their culture and identity.
- Faith communities often have a strong track record of caring for others within their local communities, including campaigning for social justice issues.
- In some areas of social work – adoption and fostering, for example – government guidelines state that workers need to be aware of, and sensitive to, the religious and spiritual needs of the children and young people whom they are placing.
- In areas of people-work, such as dealing with loss, people will often ask questions about the meaning of life which may have a religious context and undertones.
- Religion, for some people, enables them to access power and strength to make significant changes in their lives, especially when they have been going through desperate times.
- Some researchers (such as Koenig et al., 2011) are publishing studies that are beginning to show a positive correlation between faith and wellbeing; in the field of mental health, religion has been claimed to play a vital part in many people's recovery.

These are some of the factors that demonstrate how religion can impact upon people in a positive way. If this is important to the person, then you need to take it seriously as a worker, even if you do not hold a religious faith yourself.

However, you may yourself be a strong believer and belong to a faith community which informs your world view and strengthens and encourages you day by day. For you, much of the preceding discussion may feel strange, or even an example of how so many assume that people-workers will not be people of faith. There is an increasing awareness of the challenges that face people-workers of faith, to ensure that you work within your professional ethical boundaries and values yet without compromising your religious integrity, or foisting your views onto others. Much of this will emerge from completing the Activity above.

## DEALING WITH THIS IN PRACTICE

How these issues are handled can be immensely challenging. In the field of psychiatry, for example, Powell (2003) claims that, whereas some 80 per cent of patients felt that their religious and spiritual belief had a positive impact upon their illness, well over one-third of them felt unable to discuss this with their psychiatrists. This was because they feared that their beliefs would be ignored, or seen as symptoms of their illness. These professionals were giving out a very clear signal: religion is a 'no go' area as far as treatment and wellbeing are concerned, and patients quickly got the message and did not raise these topics in their consultations or interviews. A similar scenario could easily be painted for other people-work professions, including social work.

The first point to stress, therefore, is that whether you realise it or not, you will always be communicating something about your attitude towards religion when the topic crops up, even with routine form filling. If you handle it with a tick-box mentality, you will be conveying a message that, as far as you are concerned, it is of little importance. If, however, you pause at that point and ask some supplementary questions, it will at least give the other person an opportunity to say whether or not this is an important issue for them. And it will have given a message that you are open to discuss it if they wish. Supplementary questions could be something like:

'How important is your religion to you?'

'Do you attend a place of worship?'

'Do you find your faith helps you during difficult times?'

Religion can also provoke strong reactions, and you need to be aware of this. In various forms, it has contributed to human misery and oppression, and is still experienced by many people as a negative influence in the world. This is a view to which you may strongly subscribe, which may make it difficult for you to be open to different perceptions and experiences. But openness is a key feature of communication skills – you need to be able to put your own strongly held opinions and beliefs to one side, and to encourage the other person to explore issues that are important to them.

This can present difficulties, whether you have a religious faith or not. There are issues on which some faith communities appear to subscribe to a value base at odds with your professional values. There is some antagonism, for example, in some faith perspectives towards gay and lesbian relationships, and their suitability as a context for adopting children. The legal provision of civil partnerships and same-sex marriage is an affront to some religious people. In some faith communities, the position of women is at odds with how many western societies wish to celebrate equality. Jehovah's Witnesses' opposition to blood transfusions is well known, and is based upon their religious beliefs. Female genital mutilation, and male circumcision on religious grounds, are hugely emotive issues. Some workers belonging to faith communities object on principle to working with supporters of abortion. As a nurse, you may be faced with some serious personal and ethical challenges when working with a woman who is seeking an abortion, for example.

These examples have been cited because they bring to the forefront of the worker's attention some key questions which need to be asked, such as:

'Does this religious practice enrich this person's life and foster their resilience?'

'Does this religious practice in any way discriminate against anyone?'

'Does any aspect of this practice seem to be abusive in any way?'

If there seems to be discriminatory or abusive behaviour taking place, then clearly there is an obligation upon you to raise this, and find appropriate ways to challenge it. Certainly, you will need to consult your manager for advice and guidance, but to do nothing is not an option if you suspect abuse is taking place.

## Group exercise

With the help of your tutor or supervisor, explore some of the issues outlined in the previous paragraphs. What do you feel is the most appropriate response to make? Where do you draw the line between religious and cultural practices and abuse? Have you had any experiences within your own team where these issues have come to the fore? How were they dealt with? What challenges does your own faith/non-faith world view have upon your professional practice? How appropriate is it to wear a symbol of one's faith in the workplace?

## FINAL THOUGHTS

Religion and religious practice present some key challenges for people-workers, individually and as representatives of your agency. Perhaps the key questions in all such situations are these:

'To what extent does a person's religion and religious faith enrich and enhance their life, or diminish it?'

'Does their religious faith strengthen or weaken their capacity and resilience to deal with life's difficulties and tragedies?'

'To what extent does it give them a satisfying, cohesive and enriching world view?'

'Is there any evidence that there is a risk of abuse in what they are doing as a result of their religious practices?'

How you communicate with other people in this area, both verbally and non-verbally, is perhaps one of the greatest challenges to your communication skills as people-workers today.

## REFERENCES AND FURTHER READING

Canda, E. and Furman, L. (2010) *Spiritual Diversity in Social Work Practice: The Heart of Helping*, 2nd edition. New York: Oxford University Press.

Furness, S. and Gilligan, P. (2010) *Religion, Belief and Social Work: Making a Difference.* Bristol: Policy Press.

Holloway, M. and Moss, B. (2010) *Spirituality and Social Work.* Basingstoke: Palgrave Macmillan.

Koenig, H., McCullough, M. and Larson, D. (2011) *Handbook of Religion and Health*, 2nd edition. Oxford: Oxford University Press.

Moss, B. (2005) *Religion and Spirituality.* Lyme Regis: Russell House.

Powell, A. (2003) *Psychiatry and Spirituality: The Forgotten Dimension.* Brighton: Pavilion/NIMHE.

Royal College of Psychiatrists (2006) *Spirituality and Mental Health.* London: Royal College of Psychiatrists.

**RELATED CONCEPTS** anti-discriminatory practice; empathy; loss; reflective practice; spirituality

**ENGAGING WITH THE PCF** contexts and organisations; critical reflection; diversity; knowledge; values and ethics

**ENGAGING WITH THE NMC CODE** promote professionalism and trust

## Service user snippet

Marvin (32), user of mental health services:

'My faith is very important to me – I pray every day and read the scriptures and try to lead a good life … some people say I'm mad believing in God, but for me it's real, man. Just 'cos I am black and believe in God it don't mean I'm crazy … but I do want my support worker to respect my religious beliefs and not assume they are part of my illness.'

# SIMULATION

Simulation technology has become integral in the training of nurses, paramedics and operating department practitioners (ODP) for years. Mannequins can be pre-programmed to simulate breathing with a chest that can rise and fall; give birth with or without complications; bleed, vomit and display changes to their health. Students can therefore practise airway management, wound management, intravenous and advanced life support, tracheostomy care and CPR skills to name but a few, as part of their assessing, care planning and evaluating any changes in their 'patients' condition, and to develop their clinical decision making and teamworking skills.

This advanced technology provides creative challenges to other professional training programmes including social work courses. Recent studies have included the evaluation and benefits of using standardised simulation pre-programmed mannequins, and there are certainly opportunities within universities where there are shared resources within health and social care departments.

## THE JOURNEY TOWARDS SIMULATION

Many years ago student social work practical education within a classroom environment would include being pushed around in a wheelchair and to be led downstairs whilst blindfolded! The majority of practice-based learning was undertaken on placement with minimal preparation.

Role play with real or simulated service users/carers acting out a scenario then became established practice so that student social workers could have the opportunity to transfer classroom teaching into practice and develop their skills-based learning within a safe environment prior to going out on placement.

New technology has paved the way for innovations in the teaching and practising of the fundamental principles of social work or the fundamental and advanced skills of nursing, which incorporate their knowledge, value base and the transfer of theory into practice. Simulation enables nurses to practise their skills within a safe challenging environment where mistakes can be made and learnt from, without putting patients at risk. Within nursing, simulation is considered a key aspect of the pre-registration nurse education curriculum which 'supports student development through experiential learning with the opportunity for repetition, feedback, evaluation and reflection. Effective simulation facilitates safety by enhancing knowledge, behaviour and skills' (NMC, 2018: 18).

The Internet has also opened up visual pictures of what it is like to look at scenes of a person experiencing differing visual abilities and hearing different levels of deafness, but these are limited in what they actually teach.

## Activity

Research the Internet for loss of sight and hearing simulators. Although these websites will not help you fully understand how these disabilities affect a person's life, reflect on how this knowledge will support your practice.

With the development of simulation, mannequins can now be programmed to display dementia, behavioural issues, memory loss, deafness, aggression and resistance. This opens up the possibility of students assessing a 'service user mannequin' in a group; one-to-one interaction with a 'service user mannequin', or a student interacting with a 'service user mannequin' whilst being observed by their group/cohort members. With environmental technology, tutors can control the mannequins and observe via a one-way mirror as students participate in the simulation. All of this could contribute to the richness of student learning.

## TOWARDS A CRITIQUE

Whilst the technology is now available and realistic simulated environments, such as a busy hospital ward or a social work setting, can be created, can real-life aspects of relationship-based practice still be demonstrated using mannequins? Can a mannequin replace the reaction of a patient or service user/carer to a student's verbal and non-verbal communication or lack of it? Can they spontaneously ask for clarification? Can they respond to genuine warmth without making the student feel patronised? Can they replace human interaction? After all, mannequins can look eerie, and tend to be expressionless with their mouths always ajar!

### Group exercise

With the help of your tutor or supervisor, go on an exploratory fact-finding visit to a setting that uses simulation technology. This could be your local university or health setting. Consider the proposals for implementing these opportunities within your own organisation.

## FINAL THOUGHTS

As with all technology, successful integration into communication skills training for various professions will require a careful focus and evaluation of the ways in which pre-programmed mannequins might enhance the student experience in preparing them for their interactions with real people.

## REFERENCES AND FURTHER READING

Dodds, C., Heslop, P. and Meredith, C. (2018) 'Using simulation-based education to help social work students prepare for practice', *Social Work Education, The International Journal*, 37 (5): 597–602.

Logie, C., Bogo, M., Regehr, C. and Regehr, G. (2013) 'A critical appraisal of the use of standardized client simulations in social work education', *Journal of Social Work Education*, 49 (1): 66–80.

Moss, B. and Moss, S. (2019) 'It takes two to tango: simulated patients and the Clinical Skills Assessment', *InnovAiT: Education and Innovation for General Practice*, 12 (1): 18–22.

Nursing & Midwifery Council (NMC) (2018) *Realising Professionalism – Part 3: Standards for Pre-registration Nursing Programmes*. London: NMC.

**RELATED CONCEPTS** active listening; barriers to good communication; getting unstuck; non-verbal communication

**ENGAGING WITH THE PCF** skills and interventions; critical reflection and analysis

**ENGAGING WITH THE NMC CODE** practise effectively; preserve safety

### Service user snippet

Jacinda (22), nursing student:

'I was really fazed by these strange mannequin things – they seemed so, I don't know, kind of odd. But strangely once I got the hang of it it was really useful to practise stuff without fearing you would make a mistake that could hurt a real patient.'

# SOCIAL MEDIA

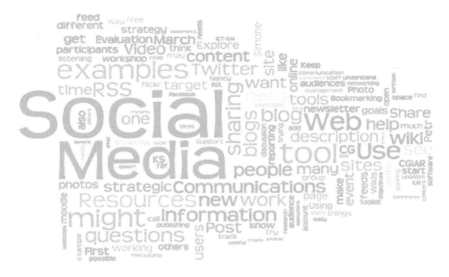

**Figure 11**  The richness and complexity of social media

'Social media' is a term used to refer to online technologies and practices that are used to share opinions and information, promote discussion and build relationships.

Twitter, Facebook, Instagram, LinkedIn, YouTube, WordPress, WhatsApp, Tumblr, Myspace, Pinterest and Flickr are just some of the array of social media tools that have rocketed over the last decade. In terms of active users per month, Twitter reports 320 million, LinkedIn over 100 million, and Facebook 1.59 billion. A report by Ofcom revealed that 83 per cent of adults use social media and 96 per cent of them have a Facebook profile. So whether you like it or not, social media is here to stay.

## Activity

Check your organisation's social media policy and raise it at a team meeting so that everyone is aware of the implications. And, of course, if you cannot find a policy or social media guidelines, start the ball rolling to develop one. Why not develop your own 'highway code'?

Many, if not most, health and social care professionals are likely to use social media for personal purposes and for social networking with family and friends. While social media can be a great tool for sharing information, it can blur the boundaries between private and professional life, so make sure that you read your organisation's social media policy. They are bound to have one, but if not, typically this will include the items shown in Table 1 later in this entry. Many professionals try to protect themselves by using a pseudonym for their social media activities in an attempt to keep a clear separation between their personal and professional lives, and find that this works well. But remember that photographs and selfies rarely lie. The best advice is to check privacy settings carefully, and consider the content. You can always try the 'granny/boss/client test', so before posting ask yourself would I want my granny/boss/client to see or read this? If in doubt, leave it out.

Much of the above guidance applies to how you, as a professional, engage with the increasingly complex array of social media. The complexity is compounded because it is so easy for the demarcation lines between the personal and the professional to become blurred. At one moment you may be contributing to a professional debate on a key issue by posting a 'tweet', and then later entertaining all your friends on Facebook with revealing photographs from your recent stag/hen party. A commitment to freedom of speech and civil liberties will recoil from any attempt at 'Big Brother' surveillance of private lives, but nevertheless you are still a professional people-worker and your commitment to your professional *persona* and reputation, as well as that of the organisation you represent, does place considerable responsibilities on your shoulders when it comes to your involvement with social media.

It is helpful at this point to see how other professionals deal with these issues. The Nursing and Midwifery Council (NMC), for example, recognises the value that social media can have for professional networking, peer support and access to ongoing learning resources. Just like other health and social care professionals, however, nurses have a responsibility to respect and maintain the confidentiality of service users and patients, and to behave in a professional manner. The NMC Code (2018) requires nurses to behave and practise in a manner that upholds the expectations and requirement of the four parts of the Code, namely:

1  Prioritise people.
2  Practise effectively.
3  Preserve safety.
4  Promote professionalism and trust.

To ensure that these professional standards are maintained, the NMC has issued social media guidance for all nurses, midwives and nursing associates. There are clear expectations here: any nurse, midwife or nursing associate who uses social media in an unprofessional manner risks the withdrawal of the registration status. Likewise, any student nurse, midwife or nursing associate who demonstrates unprofessional behaviour via social media jeopardises their entry to the professional register. All student nurses should familiarise themselves, therefore, with the NMC

*Guidance on Using Social Media Responsibly* (2019), and should also report any concerns about improper use to their tutor or supervisor.

Similarly, the Royal College of General Practitioners has developed *The Social Media Highway Code* (Riley, 2013). This is partly in response to evidence from medical students and newly qualified doctors who had viewed colleagues acting unprofessionally on Facebook; and partly because very few, if any, were aware of professional advice or guidance on how to engage with such social media. In seeking to fill this gap with the new Code, the CEO of the General Medical Council has observed that 'this is a different country, but the underlying ethics are the same … you are a professional and must retain … trust…' (Dickson, 2014).

It is worth highlighting some of the key themes from this Code (Riley, 2013) that are relevant to you as a people-work professional. These include:

1   Be aware of the image you present online and manage this proactively.
2   Recognise that the personal and professional cannot always be separated.
3   Show your human side but maintain professional boundaries.
4   Treat others with consideration, politeness and respect.
5   Remember that other people may be watching you.

Riley (2013) stresses the importance of learning how to use the privacy and profile settings of the media tools, and being aware that most social media sites do not guarantee confidentiality. He also suggests that you should only post online what you would be prepared to say in front of your grandmother or your boss, and to remember that any comments you post on social media could be quoted in other media such as the press.

## Group exercise

Within your group, Google your name to see what information *about you* pops up. How does this make you feel about the appropriateness of material being on social media and in the public domain? Is there any potential for you to feel professionally compromised by the information? As a group, draw up your own guidelines for best practice.

If you are new to social media, or setting up a social media account for work, consider using the following 'Five-Ws' based on Chambers et al. (2016):

1   Why are you using social media?
2   Which groups or people are you targeting?
3   Where will you find the groups or people you are targeting?
4   What are you hoping to achieve by using social media? What are your planned outcomes?
5   Who is going to set up and moderate the account? Who is going to train staff to use it?

## SOCIAL MEDIA DO'S AND DON'TS AT A GLANCE

Table 1 is based on Chambers et al. (2016), and outlines some helpful social media strategies.

**Table 1**  Social media strategies

| DO | DO NOT |
|---|---|
| Comply with your organisation's policies and regulations on social media. | Use email/social media to send abusive, racist or offensive messages/images. |
| Put a disclaimer on to state that your views are your own. | Disclose confidential information or client data. |
| Consider posting work-related items that will interest colleagues and share positive information. | Make disparaging comments about clients, colleagues or organisations. |
| Post items that alert colleagues to policy changes and updates. | Post anything you wouldn't show your manager/client. |
| Stop, think and consider the impact before posting. | Post work-related items on your personal account and vice versa. |

*Source*: Chambers et al. (2016)

---

### Group exercise

While there are great examples of how to use social media creatively and responsibly in health and social care, there have also been some 'casualties'. With the help of your tutor or supervisor see if you can discover examples within your own profession(s) where the unprofessional use of social media has led to disciplinary proceedings being taken.

---

## FINAL THOUGHTS

Social media programs are constantly developing, with new platforms and new opportunities emerging. How you and your organisation(s) respond will be important as you seek to maintain your core professional values.

## REFERENCES AND FURTHER READING

Chambers, R., Schmid, M. and Birch-Jones, J. (2016) *Digital Healthcare: The Essential Guide*. Oxford: Otmoor.

Dickson, N. (2014) Cited in a conference presentation by Dr Ben Riley (RCGPs) on the *Social Media Highway Code*. Keele University Medical School, 23 March.

Nursing & Midwifery Council (NMC) (2018) *The Code: Professional Standards of Practice and Behaviour for Nurses, Midwives and Nursing Associates.* London: NMC.

Nursing & Midwifery Council (NMC) (2019) *Guidance on Using Social Media Responsibly.* London: NMC. Available at www.nmc.org.uk/globalassets/sitedocuments/nmc-publica tions/social-media-guidance.pdf (accessed 24/10/19).

Novell, R.J. (2013) 'Social workers should use social media to challenge public perceptions', *Guardian*, 23 July. Available at www.theguardian.com/social-care-network/2013/jul/23/ social-workers-social-media-challenge-perception (accessed 15/10/19).

Ofcom (The Central Office of Information) (2009) 'Engaging through Social Media'. Available at www.ofcom.org.uk/social networking (accessed 11/09/19)

Riley, B. (2013) *The Social Media Highway Code.* London: Royal College of General Practitioners. Available at www.rcgp.org.uk/social-media (accessed 15/10/19).

**RELATED CONCEPTS** confidentiality; establishing a professional relationship; information technology (ICT) and health informatics

**ENGAGING WITH THE PCF** professionalism; values and ethics; context and organisation; personal leadership

**ENGAGING WITH THE NMC CODE** promote professionalism and trust

### Service user snippet

Josh (19):

'I so nearly got my fingers badly burned by putting some obscene material onto my Facebook page as a joke. I changed my mind at the last minute – thank goodness I did. I could have been thrown off my course.'

# SPIRITUALITY

There is a growing interest in spirituality in contemporary society, evidenced by a burgeoning bookshop trade in alternative therapies, meditation techniques, 'new age' religions, and what seems like 1,001 ways in which to find peace and fulfilment in an increasingly frenetic western society. The appeal of various eastern mystic and spiritual traditions is increasing, and many religious groups are experiencing a surge of interest as some traditional forms of religion seem to be in rapid decline.

As a concept, however, spirituality is notoriously difficult to define. For faith communities spirituality reflects their religious and devotional practices, such as prayer, meditation and worship. Spirituality points them towards a deeper 'divine' mystery, a sense of awe, wonder and beauty. It also can motivate them to serve and care for others and struggle for social justice.

If, by contrast, you ask someone with no religious faith, they may respond with ideas of 'wellbeing', meaning and purpose, and whatever enriches life and makes it worth living. They too may refer to mystery, awe and wonder, but without any 'divine' or 'otherworldly' connotations. They too will seek to care for others and improve society by challenging injustice. Spirituality therefore may be seen to be a 'signposting' or 'gateway' word that has a range of meanings across a wide spectrum, but which nevertheless has some common features.

The significance of all of this for your communication skills as people-workers and especially as nurses is that you will often find yourself engaging at quite a deep level with people, especially at times of crisis and loss. Such momentous events in people's lives often evoke the unanswerable questions of 'why': 'Why should this happen to me?', 'Why does God allow this to happen?', 'What have I done to deserve this?'. Such inchoate and painful outpourings are not easy to respond to with integrity. Your role is not to offer 'answers', but you are likely to share the other person's distress. So you need to think about the communication skills that are necessary in such situations.

The 'territory' to which spirituality points seems to have some or all of the following features:

- People's need to feel somehow connected to something wider or 'beyond'.
- A sense that something is missing in their lives: a feeling of emptiness, and being without hope or purpose in life.
- A sense of not being of value – of not mattering to anyone.
- Feelings of being hurt or damaged in some way.

- People's sense that life has let them down, and they have not got what they deserve.
- Feelings of guilt.
- The need to make some sense of life, and to find a world view that is sufficiently satisfying to deal with the mess, as well as the glory, of living.
- Questions about where people draw their strength from, especially in times of need.
- Questions about who or what, if anything, is 'in control'.
- Questions about what they are going to do with their life.
- Questions and worries about what happens after death.

These are some of the difficult areas of human living that prompt questions about spirituality when a previous world view is disturbed or even shattered. *We thought we had the measure of things, but now this has happened, we are not so sure – and it hurts.*

The other side of the coin is when someone's world view proves sufficiently durable, flexible and resilient to absorb such painful questions and to remain intact; it then gives them greater strength to cope even when awful 'unanswerable' things happen.

## SOME GUIDELINES TO CONSIDER

- *Being, not doing*: When people are feeling in touch with these profound and at times often distressing feelings, it is comforting for you simply to be there with them. Sometimes it helps the other person just to know their space is being shared for a while, to ease their aloneness.
- *Asking, not telling*: It is so tempting to offer answers to what in the end are unanswerable questions. It makes us feel better. But even if our responses satisfy us, there is no guarantee that they will satisfy the other person.
- *Going with the flow, not forcing the agenda*: It is more important to let the other person dictate the speed at which your interview or discussion flows. Sometimes important unexpected issues may emerge in the middle of a session that you have carefully prepared and timed. Resist the temptation to get the interview back on track: you will be more helpful if you let them explore their difficult feelings and reactions.
- *Being humble and not a 'know-all'*: All professional people-workers are in some ways experts, and it is one of the pleasures of the job sometimes to be able to use that expertise in effective and appropriate ways. With spirituality, however, none of us is expert enough to provide answers for other people. Instead, we all have to find our way through this complicated territory. Your role as people-workers in such situations is to share others' journey as companionably as possible. This involves stepping back from your own expertise and being open and humble enough to let people find their own way with whatever support you are able to offer as a fellow traveller.

## SOME HELPFUL APPROACHES

There are some helpful questions and comments you can ask the person in turmoil who is trying to make sense of what is happening to them. These may include:

'J, in what ways is all of this difficult for you to get your head around? Does all of this make you wonder what it is all about, J?'

'Do you think, J, that there is someone or something who is supposed to be running the show?'

'Do you think that somehow it has all gone wrong?'

'J, do you ever try to pray when you run into difficulties?'

'How did you see your world, J, before all this happened? How is it different now? Do you think, J, that there is a higher power we can turn to in some ways?'

'How do you normally handle things when they go wrong, J? Whom do you tend to turn to, J, when you need help and support?'

'Do you believe in fate, J? Do you read your horoscope? Do you believe it?'

None of these questions is foolproof. The most important thing is to find your own authentic style in such situations, so that you are being the 'real you'. You need to be able to communicate to the other person that you are concerned for them, that you are not going to give them a set of glib, easy answers, and that, as far as you can, you are willing to share some of their journey with them. To be able to communicate those messages is the real skill: it speaks volumes about your shared humanity, and is an approach that may be far more empowering than you ever realise.

## Activity

Are you able to identify situations in your own or other people's lives, where issues of spirituality have been raised or hinted at? What were the underlying issues and concerns? How were you able to respond?

## SPIRITUAL INTELLIGENCE

Another significant contribution to this debate has been made by Zohar and Marshall (1999), who have added the concept of spiritual intelligence (SQ) to the existing theoretical frameworks of IQ and emotional intelligence. By using this concept of SQ, these writers encourage us to see a spiritual dimension in ourselves and in others, and offer some core indicators that have strong connections to people-work practice. These include:

- The capacity to be flexible.
- A high degree of self-awareness.
- A capacity to face and use suffering.
- A capacity to face and transcend pain.
- The quality of being inspired by vision and values.

The concept of SQ brings another strand of meaning and richness to this theme of spirituality.

## Group exercise

With the help of your tutor or supervisor, explore in your group the issues raised in this chapter. Be honest about your reactions, positive, negative or puzzled! In what ways do you think that your own practice might be enriched by an understanding and awareness of these issues?

## FINAL THOUGHTS

If you feel uncomfortable dealing with difficult issues, the temptation to run away is strong, thereby allowing your own discomfort to determine the agenda. This theme of spirituality challenges you to clarify your own world view and how satisfying it is, especially during your times of crisis. Spirituality therefore is the journey of being human, and what makes us tick. Every now and again you will be privileged to share this with another person in their moments of pain. To flinch from that privilege would not only let the other person down; in doing so, you would be letting yourself down too.

## REFERENCES AND FURTHER READING

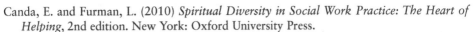

Canda, E. and Furman, L. (2010) *Spiritual Diversity in Social Work Practice: The Heart of Helping*, 2nd edition. New York: Oxford University Press.
Dudley, J. (2019) *Spiritual Meditations for People Who Help Other People*. Botsford, CT: North American Association of Christians in Social Work (NACSW).
Holloway, M. and Moss, B. (2010) *Spirituality and Social Work*. Basingstoke: Palgrave Macmillan.
Mathews, I. (2009) *Social Work and Spirituality*. Exeter: Learning Matters.
McSherry, W. (2006) *Making Sense of Spirituality in Nursing and Healthcare Practice: An Interactive Approach*, 2nd edition. London: Jessica Kingsley.
Moss, B. (2005) *Religion and Spirituality*. Lyme Regis: Russell House.
Zohar, D. and Marshall, I. (1999) *SQ: Connecting with our Spiritual Intelligence*. London: Bloomsbury.

**RELATED CONCEPTS** anti-discriminatory practice; establishing a professional relationship; reflective practice; religion

**ENGAGING WITH THE PCF** diversity; professionalism; skills and interventions; values and ethics

**ENGAGING WITH THE NMC CODE** prioritise people; promote professionalism and trust

---

### Service user snippet

Jennifer (25), nurse:

'I wouldn't call myself religious but I have this deep sense of there being something more to life ... I can't put it into words but when I started to read some of the course books on spirituality it kind of made sense and I could see how important it is for everyone, and that it is somehow part of the whole.'

# SUICIDE

One of the most challenging scenarios facing any people-worker is the person who is feeling so deeply desperate that they don't think there is any point in carrying on. They are caught up in a maelstrom of conflicting emotions, and often feel they are sinking slowly into oblivion where no one can help because no one cares. Without doubt, it is uniquely challenging and scary for any people-worker to be faced with someone for whom the prospect of carrying on living or facing a dark and uncertain future is unbearable. Often the people-worker mirrors a similar sense of helplessness: *What can I do? What can I say? How can I make a difference? Upon what resources can I draw to deal with this so painful situation?*

## Activity

Find out where your local branch of the Samaritans is located. Get in touch with them so that you are aware of the help and support they can give to desperate and suicidal people. Obtain some of their contact literature so that you can have it to hand when needed.

Obviously, the exact circumstances in which you find yourself will impact upon how you seek to handle such difficult situations. Unless you are in an urgent life-or-death scenario where emergency services need to be called, there is one useful rule of thumb to keep firmly in mind when working with someone who is feeling suicidal. You may be the nurse at the bedside of a patient to has tried to take their own life and is the first person they see when they come round. How you respond will be so important.

This is best expressed in Neil Thompson's famous dictum: *what this person needs is a good listening to!* In other words, the most important gift we can offer to someone who is feeling at the end of their tether is our time and undivided attention. *Don't just do something – be there* is another way of putting it. Concentrated compassionate listening is not easy, but it can be liberating and life-affirming for someone who may be feeling unloved, unnoticed and marginalised.

Inevitably, when faced with someone overwhelmed by negative feelings, we may struggle to know how best to engage with them sensitively, including the delicate issue of assessing how serious they are about ending their lives. A calm, gentle approach could include asking some or all of the following questions about a person's suicidal thoughts:

'Some people in situations like yours, J, may wonder if it is worth carrying on ... or even ending it all.' (*Note*: this is a 'normalising' and relatively unthreatening question that may help the person feel that this can be shared territory.)

'Can I ask you, J, have you ever thought about ending your life?'

If the response to this is 'yes', then there are some helpful follow-up questions you could use such as:

'When you are thinking in this way, J, have you got as far as devising a plan for how you would end your life?'

'Are you able to tell me how detailed your plan is?'

'How easy would it be to put that plan into action?'

'When do you think you might do it?'

It is also important to explore what protective measures may be in place that would make the person hesitate before taking their own life. For example:

'Is there anything or anyone who would stop you from doing this, J?'

'What is important to you in your life?'

'Is there anyone who is especially close to you?'

'Who do you think would miss you most?'

'What are your happiest memories?'

Clearly the outcome of such a discussion will depend on how the person responds to your caring questioning. You will soon gain a clear picture of how desperate the person really is. Take comfort from the fact that they trust you enough to disclose such intimate and painful information, and that to some degree at least they have placed their lives into your caring hands.

Your next task will be to work out together what happens next: whether the situation is so serious that you need to obtain immediate medical or psychiatric help; whether a further contact/appointment is possible; where they are living and how to contact them again. You may well need to take advice from your manager or another colleague while the person is still with you, either face to face or by ringing them up.

## Group exercise

With the help of your tutor or supervisor, discuss any scenarios you are aware of that have involved suicide. What guidelines does your organisation suggest to help you deal with such situations? What duty of care does your organisation have towards those who deal with such distressing situations?

## FINAL THOUGHTS

Whatever the outcome you will feel pretty churned up by the experience, so it is important that you offload your worries and anxieties to a colleague or supervisor as soon as you can, and, if appropriate, record what has happened in your agency records.

## REFERENCES AND FURTHER READING

Durkheim, E. (2006) *On Suicide*. London: Penguin.
Phelan, H. (2018) 'How to talk to a suicidal patient', *Nursing Times*, 20 June.
Pomphrey, S. (2011) 'Suicide – personally and professionally', *Social Work Today*, 11 (5): 6ff.

### Web resources

Mental Health Foundation, general website – www.mentalhealth.org.uk (accessed 15/10/19)
Mental Health Foundation, Suicide – www.mentalhealth.org.uk/a-to-z/s/suicide (accessed 15/10/19)

**RELATED CONCEPTS** breaking bad news; empathy; reflective practice; religion; spirituality; whistleblowing

**ENGAGING WITH THE PCF** skills and interventions; professionalism; values and ethics

**ENGAGING WITH THE NMC CODE** preserve safety; promote professionalism and trust

### Service user snippet

Seb (31), former Marine:

'I never thought I would get so low after my discharge from the Marines. I lost everything and felt I had nothing to live for and nowhere to turn. I felt so ashamed. I stood on the railway bridge waiting to jump … and if it hadn't been for an off-duty nurse who came up to me, asked how I was, and gave some time to me, I think I would have jumped. I really do. I owe my life to her.'

# SUPERVISION

Many people-workers have mixed feelings about supervision. They agree with the rhetoric about its importance, but often report that the reality is quite different, with sessions that are more tokenistic than being really helpful to develop and sustain best practice. As Thompson (2006: 75) notes:

> Some people see it primarily or even exclusively as a means of ensuring that sufficient quality and quantity of work is being carried out – what is often referred to as 'snoopervision'.

Supervision for people-workers is nevertheless essential for the following reasons:

- It provides a context in which you can be supported and encouraged.
- It provides the structure for accountability to be maintained and exercised, as your work is scrutinised and evaluated. But it is not a performance audit, that should happen at another occasion.
- It provides an opportunity for your learning and your critical skills to be explored and improved.
- It provides opportunities for your continuing professional development (CPD) to be discussed and planned, especially for professional re-registration.

Supervision gives expression to the central tenet of people-work, that it is a shared responsibility; you do not have to soldier on alone or in isolation. It also reinforces the basic principle that in doing your work, you are a representative of the agency that employs you, and are fundamentally accountable for the work you undertake.

It is no coincidence that the importance of supervision has come under increasing scrutiny following major scandals involving child sexual abuse and the Mid Staffordshire NHS Trust, where the quality of care has been seriously, even tragically, compromised (Francis, 2013). In their review of the importance of supervision, Morrison and Wonnacott (2010: 1) draw attention to Lord Laming's insistence that 'social work is carried out in a supportive learning environment that actively encourages the continuous development of professional judgement and skills. Regular high quality organized supervision is critical.' Morrison and Wonnacott (2010: 1) observe that until the publication of *Providing Effective Supervision* (CWDC/Skills for Care, 2007) there had been little national attention given to creating robust policy frameworks and that *too often we settle for having supervision rather than having good supervision* – a crucial difference. Furthermore, Lord Laming's (2009: 32) trenchant critique will hold true for many different aspects of people-work: 'individuals are carrying too much personal responsibility with no outlet for the sometimes severe emotional and psychological stresses that staff … often face.' This need for organisations to provide high-quality supervision has been further strengthened by: (1) the work of Eileen Munro (2011) who laments the managerial emphasis upon performance that leaves little time for thoughtful consideration; (2) the development of the former College of Social Work; and (3) Morrison's (2005) work on developing an integrated model for supervision that takes into account organisational and interagency aspects of the supervisory process.

## Activity

Think about some experiences you have had of supervision. What has worked well for you? What are the hallmarks of good supervision? Have you had instances of poor supervision? How did these experiences make you feel?

There are several books you can read to explore supervision in depth, but here are some of the key points you need to bear in mind, whether you are the supervisor or supervisee:

- Be well prepared; know why you are meeting and the issues you need to talk about, and be open to each of you contributing to the final agenda.
- Agree the date, time and venue for the meeting; be sure to keep the appointment. In an extreme emergency, consult your supervisor (in advance, if possible) to re-schedule your session.
- Decide what room layout best meets your needs.
- Ensure that you are not disturbed. Inform the receptionist(s) and ask them not to put any calls through to you. Switch off your mobile phone and/or pager.

All of these points help you communicate clearly that you are taking supervision seriously and want to make the very best of the time you have together. This involves being:

- *Assertive*: You need to know what the supervision session should be achieving. If this is not happening, you need to say so, firmly but politely, and ask for specific issues to be addressed. Do not leave the session smouldering with resentment that key issues have not been tackled.
- *Open and reflective*: Your work is about how you interact with people and how they respond. Supervision, therefore, will often entail personal scrutiny, and unless you are willing to engage with that process you will not be able to improve your practice. Remember that critical appraisal of your performance is just that: a critique of your *performance*. It is not a personal attack. The best workers are always keen to learn how to improve.
- *Responsive*: This flows from being reflective. Supervision is an opportunity for real dialogue. It is not a one-way process. This does not mean that you will

always agree with what the other person says: a frank exchange of opposing views can become extraordinarily insightful at times. But always seek to develop the skill of showing responsiveness so that it is clear that you are committed to improving your practice. If you allow yourself to become defensive and put barriers up, then you will be letting yourself down.

- *Accurate*: Whether you are seeking to explain some aspect of your work, or are recording the notes from your supervision session afterwards, always seek to be accurate, truthful and honest. It may be difficult at times to admit to giving a poor level of service to someone, or to allowing certain feelings to cloud your judgement, but an admission and discussion of these will help to ensure that you do better next time.

## A NOTE OF CAUTION

To some of you, these guidelines may feel utopian because your experience of supervision has either been non-existent or you have been supervised by a line manager in whom you place very little trust. Indeed, you may suspect that if you tell things 'as they really are' you may receive less rather than more support, or even be 'cold-shouldered' or punished in some way. You may even fear that promotion opportunities, and future references, may be put in jeopardy. This can be a real 'double-bind', and it would be naive to suggest that there is an easy answer.

Some suggestions are worth considering, however, to see if you can improve the quality and usefulness of your supervision sessions. For example:

- Share your concerns with another colleague whom you can trust; see if they have had similar experiences.
- Write a note to your supervisor before your next session, offering items for the agenda, specifically asking for a discussion on issues you wish to raise.
- In the session itself, take the initiative to raise such issues. You will want to choose these carefully, of course, if you are feeling uneasy about exposing your vulnerability.
- Check your job description and agency policies to see what mention is made of supervision and the expectations of supervision.
- Raise the matter tactfully in a team meeting to see if there are ways in which, as a team, supervision can be made more rewarding for everyone concerned.
- You may wish to consider raising your issues informally with a member of the senior management team, or your union representative, to see what can be done.
- If all of this fails, you may wish to consider using the complaints procedure so that the senior management of the agency is made aware of your concerns.
- As a last resort, you need to be asking yourself if this is really the kind of agency you should be working for. Maybe the time has come to look for something else.

In all the suggested approaches outlined above, your communication skills and tactfulness will be fully tested. Think carefully about how you will broach these issues, and ensure that you do so in a calm, professional manner. Keep notes of everything you do and say, and of all the responses you receive.

## NURSING PERSPECTIVES

Within nursing, clinical supervision is a key component of developing professional practice to ensure high-quality patient care. Through reflection and discussion of concerns and experiences with a tutor or supervisor, new perspectives can be developed. The process of clinical supervision can help you to feel supported, reduce your stress levels and help you gain new insights. By furthering your learning and understanding you will be able to develop confidence and competence in your clinical skills and clinical decision-making abilities.

As a qualified nurse you will be expected to reflect on your practice and professional development regularly. During your revalidation process you will need to evidence your reflections and discuss your learning and any areas for further development during your reflective discussion with another NMC registrant. The revalidation process is an important part of ensuring that your professional practice is up to date, and that you are conforming to all four parts of the NMC Code, namely: (1) Prioritise people; (2) Practise effectively; (3) Preserve safety; (4) Promote professionalism and trust.

## GROUP SUPERVISION

Many agencies, especially those heavily involved with training newly qualified or student workers, will make use of group supervision as part of the supervisory relationship. How this works in practice may vary depending on the supervisor. But of the four functions of supervision mentioned at the outset, only two are really appropriate for group supervision, namely discussion of the work being undertaken, and the teaching and development of the knowledge and skills needed for the work. Although group supervision can be enormously encouraging and supportive for everyone concerned, anything that is specifically personal to an individual should not be raised in a group session, but should be kept for one-to-one supervision. Concern for appropriate confidentiality, in other words, should be high on the agenda.

Group discussions require a certain discipline and a willingness to follow ground rules so that everyone can contribute and benefit. The communication skills or 'rules' necessary for successful group supervision include:

- Don't interrupt when someone else is talking.
- Don't 'hog the show'; be brief and to the point when talking yourself.
- Be willing to take part – do not sit in silence and let others do all the work.
- Remember that you will have useful things to contribute to help others learn, as well as gaining benefit from listening to them.
- Encourage reticent members to participate: remember that some people do find it quite difficult to speak up in front of a group.

- Don't be afraid to ask questions. It is easy to feel reticent in front of others, and to feel a little foolish asking about what you think you will be expected to know already. Remember, though, that there should be no such thing as a 'silly question', and that for everyone who asks the question there will be several more who will be grateful that they have done so.
- Keep to the agreed time for discussions, and keep to the point.
- Respect the group leader, who from time to time may need to move the discussion forward, even if you don't feel ready to do so.
- Find ways of ensuring that your needs are met. If for any reason you leave the meeting with unresolved issues, make a careful note of them and raise them with your supervisor next time you meet, or send a note asking for time to discuss your issues further. This is all about taking responsibility for your own learning.
- Group leaders, of course, have a specific responsibility to ensure that the group keeps to the agreed tasks, and that dominant members do not take over the discussion to the detriment of others. But it is also up to group members to be keen to contribute and to challenge anyone who is behaving inappropriately.

## Group exercise

With the help of your tutor or supervisor, work together in small groups to draw up a group learning agreement for a forthcoming multi-agency support group involving students from several different disciplines. *Topic*: Continuing professional development – how can we support each other as a multi-professional group of learners?

## FINAL THOUGHTS

Insisting on good supervision, whether you are the supervisor or supervisee, is part of your core commitment to best practice. It is a defined mechanism for taking good care of yourself professionally so that you can deliver better outcomes. Good supervision, therefore, is what you, and they, and your organisation deserve.

## REFERENCES AND FURTHER READING

CWDC/Skills for Care (2007) *Providing Effective Supervision: Effective Workforce Development Tool*. Leeds: CWDC/Skills for Care.

Francis, R. (2013) *Report of the Mid Staffordshire NHS Foundation Trust Public Inquiry*. Norwich: TSO.

Hawkins, P. and Shohet, R. (2012) *Supervision in the Helping Professions*, 4th edition. Buckingham: Open University Press.

Laming, H. (2009) *The Protection of Children in England*. Norwich: TSO.

Morrison, T. (2005) *Staff Supervision in Social Care: Making a Real Difference to Staff and Service Users*, 3rd edition. Brighton: Pavilion.

Morrison, T. and Wonnacott, J. (2010) 'Supervision: now or never – reclaiming reflective supervision in social work', In-Trac, February. Available at In-trac.co.uk/supervision-now-or-never (accessed 23/02/17).

Munro, E. (2011) *The Munro Review of Child Protection: Final Report – A Child Centred System*, CM 8062. Norwich: TSO.

Nursing & Midwifery Council (NMC) (2018) *Future Nurse: Standards of Proficiency for Registered Nurses*. London: NMC.

Thompson, N. (2006) *Promoting Workplace Learning*. Bristol: The Policy Press.

Thompson, N. (2012) *The People Solutions Sourcebook*, 2nd edition. Basingstoke: Palgrave Macmillan.

Thompson, N. and Gilbert, P. (2011) *Supervision Skills: A Learning and Development Manual*. Lyme Regis: Russell House.

**RELATED CONCEPTS** confidentiality; feedback (giving and receiving); reflective practice

**ENGAGING WITH THE PCF** context and organisations; critical reflection; professional leadership; values and ethics

**ENGAGING WITH THE NMC CODE** promote professionalism and trust

### Service user snippet

Jaycee (23), recently qualified social worker:

'You hear all these horror stories about rubbish supervision or managers not being bothered to give it, but I can honestly say that everyone in my new team really looks forward to supervision and finds it really useful in our stressful jobs. OK, we may be the exception, but I thank my lucky stars that supervision works for me.'

# TALKS AND PRESENTATIONS

It is becoming increasingly important for people-workers to be able to prepare and deliver good quality talks and presentations. This will sometimes be in your job description; it is often part of the selection process for getting the job in the first place. Good quality communication skills are essential, and time spent on practising and improving these skills will work wonders both for your confidence and your effectiveness as a communicator.

---

## Activity

Make a list of the occasions and opportunities both within your agency and beyond, where talks and presentations are needed from time to time. These can range from very low-key, informal talks involving a small number of colleagues, to more formal 'set piece' occasions.

Think of some of the talks and presentations you have attended. What marks out the good ones from the mediocre or poor ones? Note these points down and keep them to hand to refer to in the discussion that follows.

---

The skills you need to deliver a good talk or presentation are not in themselves difficult, but attention must be given to them if you are to succeed. When you listen to a good speaker, it all seems to be effortless, but in order to reach that standard, a lot of work has to be done by way of preparation.

There are three things you need to know: your audience and its context, your material, and your limitations.

## KNOWING YOUR AUDIENCE AND ITS CONTEXT

Knowing your audience is vitally important. Talking to senior managers or a group of young students will demand different approaches. So you need to know in advance:

- Who exactly will be there?
- What do they want to know about?
- What level of knowledge can you assume they already have?
- What is the title and topic of the talk?

- How long do they want you to talk for?
- Will there be questions and discussion to follow?
- Are you the only speaker? Have others been invited to talk about other topics?
- What is the unique contribution you can make?
- What is the venue like? Is it a formal or informal setting?
- Who will act as convenor/chair of the meeting? Can you talk to them in advance to help you in your preparation?
- What visual aid/PowerPoint/internet access facilities are there?
- Will the organisation require you to submit your PowerPoint presentation in advance? They may not allow you to use your memory stick on the day because of security/virus protection issues.
- Do they need a digest or summary in advance of the meeting?
- Are you expected to provide handouts? If so, who will provide enough copies for everyone?
- What is the 'dress code' for the occasion?
- Are expenses/fees paid? If you are doing this as part of your work, how will this be negotiated?
- What permissions will you need from your agency to undertake this work?
- Will you know anyone in the audience, or is it likely to be a complete 'sea of strangers'?
- How much time do you need to prepare for this event? Do you need to negotiate this with your manager?
- Is there a lectern or desk for you to put your notes on?
- How will you get feedback afterwards? Will they welcome a feedback sheet being provided for them to complete and return to you?

This may seem, at first, to be a bewildering set of questions and issues to tackle in advance, but if you reflect carefully on them you will begin to appreciate that the answers you receive to each of them are an important part of the preparation jigsaw. Importantly, this information will help you feel more assured and well prepared by reducing the 'areas of the unknown'. The more you feel in charge of things, the more confident you are likely to be.


## KNOW YOUR MATERIAL

Perhaps you have been to meetings where an ill-prepared speaker mumbles, constantly shuffling through a sheaf of notes, unable to communicate effectively with you as an audience. You most definitely do not want to be like that! And you won't be, *if* you follow some basic guidelines in your preparation. These include:

- Survey the range of issues and information relevant to the subject. Spend time selecting the most appropriate material.
- Decide what can be done within the time. Clearly, if you are giving an overview of a subject for 15 minutes, you can only briefly highlight three or four main themes. If you have an hour, then you need to decide whether to go wider or

deeper. You could keep to the same three or four points and say a lot more about each one or you could increase the themes you cover to seven or eight. In some ways, only you can decide this, but it may help to discuss the possibilities with the person who is running the meeting to see what they think would be most helpful.

- Think about how you can bring the subject to life. Are there stories you can tell which illustrate the themes you are covering? These must, of course, be totally anonymised, but the human 'slant' often helps to bring a topic to life and capture the attention of the audience.

- What visual aids will support your talk? If you are using PowerPoint, remember the golden rule about not putting too much information on any one slide. Ensure that your slides are clear, succinct and meet current guidelines. Think about what the audience will find most helpful.

- Having chosen your material, decide in what order you wish to present your chosen topics and how much time to give to each theme. Is there a particular 'take' or approach that will help the audience to remember what you are saying? A real-life (anonymised) story, for instance, or some topical reference, can enliven your presentation.

- What 'memory props' will you need? Most speakers need to refer to some sort of 'comfort pad' for their notes. Try to get the balance right between referring to notes or even the full-length script, and actually talking to the audience. The more you can maintain eye contact with the audience, the more effective your talk will be. But only the most experienced can deliver a talk from memory. And even they can 'dry up' sometimes and find that their minds go blank – so you do need to have notes easily to hand. You need to decide what will work best for you, and then prepare fully.

- Some people use a set of small cards just for the main points, or have the main headings on their tablet or laptop. Whatever works for you is fine, but remember to write large and clear: in the heat of the moment, you need to read what you have written at a glance.

- Rehearse your talk – by yourself and with a supportive friend. This serves several purposes. It begins to give you the 'feel' of delivering the material and making it your own. You will begin to develop your own personal style and gain confidence. It will also test out the time it takes to deliver the talk. You do not want to run out of things to say with five minutes left for you to fill, or to find that you have entered 'injury time' with only a few minutes left, when you are only half way through your material. You will be surprised in your early days of giving talks about how little, or how long, it takes to deliver your material. Clearly, you should not rattle through the talk at breakneck speed in order to get the most information across. You will lose people in the first 30 seconds if you do that. Nor should you adopt a slow, laborious and heavy style that makes five minutes feel like an eternity. Try to be your usual self with a conversational style, but vary the speed of the delivery to maintain interest. Remember that an audience's attention span can be quite limited, so break up your talk into easily identified sections and chunks.

- Practise using the PowerPoint slides as background so that you are comfortable with the technology.

- Humour can be a good communication skill to use, but be careful. Use it sparingly, and ensure that it is appropriate to the occasion and that you can deliver it confidently. A humorous story or joke that goes down like a lead balloon is counter-productive and can be difficult to recover from.
- Think about the 'music' of your voice. Whatever the content of your talk, your vocal delivery will make or break it. A monotonous delivery will quickly lose the audience, for whom it will feel like a recitation from the telephone directory. By contrast, too 'sing-song' a delivery can be jarring and off-putting. Try to be natural, but to use as much variation in your tone, pitch and speed of delivery as possible.

---

## Activity

Listen to the professionals on television or radio news bulletins. Listen not so much to *what* they are saying but *how* they say it. Close your eyes as you listen to them. Very rarely will they deliver two or three words together on the same 'note' (as in musical notes). There will be subtle variations in the pace of delivery in order to maintain your interest. That is what you are aiming at!

Record your talk – or part of it – and then listen to yourself, and see how you can improve the 'music' of your spoken delivery.

---

## KNOW YOUR LIMITATIONS

You can get quite a buzz from a well-delivered, well-received talk or presentation. By contrast, if you have tried to be too ambitious, or have used complicated visual aids that have not worked well, you can quickly feel deflated. In the early days, therefore, try not to overstretch yourself or be too ambitious. A simple, straightforward talk that is well prepared and well delivered will always go down well; someone who tries to be a 'clever clogs' is likely to lose the sympathy of the audience.

## ON THE DAY ITSELF

However well prepared you are, you will still feel nervous about the occasion. Believe it or not, this is to be welcomed! It means you are taking the event seriously. Anyone giving a performance, even 'old hands', will say that nervousness beforehand is an essential ingredient for ensuring that the adrenalin flows to help you give your best.

Some useful tips include the following:

- Ensure that you know exactly where you have to go, and arrive in good time.
- On arrival, look for the person in charge to let them know you are there.
- Check the layout of the room and see whether you need to make any adjustments to the furniture. You do not want to be totally hidden by a huge lectern or

reading desk, or to find that there is nowhere to put your notes to enable you to refer to them easily.

- Check the equipment you will be using. If you have brought your own laptop and projector, check that it works, and set it up in good time. If you are using their equipment, ensure that you are comfortable with how to use it. If you have sent your material through in advance, check that it is on the system and ready to use. Do not be afraid to ask for help! This is another reason for arriving early, so that everything can be ready to start on time.

- If you plan to access the Internet during your presentation, double-check that this is possible and that you can access the material or the video-clip easily. Signal failure can thwart even the best prepared presentation.

- Check whether there is a public address (PA) system and whether you will need to use a microphone. If so, is this on an adjustable stand, or clipped to your lapel, or a hand-held 'lollypop'? Make yourself familiar with it, and check the voice level before the meeting so that you know how best to speak. Remember that good PA systems work best if you use your normal speaking voice, but some of the equipment you encounter may need to be tamed in advance! PA systems are also important for people who use hearing aids, so do not get into the habit of offhandedly refusing to use it or saying that you do not need it, or do not like to use it. Other people may well need it, and you must be sensitive to their needs. The hand-held 'lollypop' microphones can pose an additional hazard, of course, especially if you are using other visual aids or working your laptop. Spend a few moments getting things in the right place on the table. Maybe you will need to ask someone else to operate the laptop for you in order to have at least one hand free.

- Many people like to have a glass of water to hand. Do ask if one is not already available on the table for you.

- Check the order of proceedings and where you should sit before you are called to speak.

- Double-check your notes and everything you need.

- If you are offering a brief feedback sheet for the audience to complete afterwards, ask the chair if you can distribute them beforehand on seats. This saves you forgetting, or having to hand them out in a rush afterwards.

## WHAT TO DO ABOUT HANDOUTS

You will need to decide what approach to adopt in regard to handouts, assuming of course that you have prepared some. There are two schools of thought about handouts: give them out at the beginning, or give them out at the end. There are advantages (+) and pitfalls (−) with each approach, and you need to decide which will work best for you.

### Giving them out in advance

+ People can see the points you are making and have the overview at their fingertips.

+ They can make their own notes on the handout, especially if it adopts the PowerPoint layout with space for notes against each slide.
+ You can add complex information, charts, diagrams, pictures and quotations that you can refer to during the talk, and ask people to read, more easily than putting such complex information on a screen in front of them.
- People are likely to jump ahead and look for what you are going to say, rather than concentrating on the actual talk.
- People will study the handout, and you have the riveting prospect of talking to a sea of bowed heads.
- People often drop them during the talk and scrabble around noisily to retrieve them.
- Handouts invite people to use them as scribble pads for purposes which have nothing to do with your talk.

## Giving them out afterwards

+ People do not have a paper-based distraction. They can focus all their attention on you and what you are saying.
+ You have some greater flexibility in how you deliver your material. If you do not stick slavishly to the order of the material as laid down in the handout, no one will know, whereas if they are following your points and you deviate from them, they may start checking nervously with each other.
- People do like to have the chance to make their own notes, and to jot down their questions and comments as the talk proceeds; a handout stimulates this process.
- Some like to use a handout to do some lateral multi-task thinking about the issues you raise.

The choice is yours, and it may be a case of trial and error for the first few occasions. If you do decide to give them out at the end, then it is important to let people know this at the beginning.

Another solution would be to upload them onto the organiser's website afterwards, if this is available to you.

# GETTING ONTO YOUR FEET

Once you are called forward, the following golden rules will stand you in good stead:

• Stand comfortably in front of your audience, and generally keep still. A fidgety speaker, who rocks to and fro, or who makes unnecessary movements can be distracting. After you have given several talks, you will develop your own style that may involve some modest movement, but unless you do it well it can be distracting.
• Before you utter a single word, look at the audience and give them a smile. This communicates a welcoming approach from you, and immediately begins to

engage your audience. You need to try to make that essential human connection between yourself and the audience from the word 'go', and a smile is a great way to begin to do that.

- It is often appropriate to begin by thanking the chair for the invitation. You may wish to add that you feel honoured and privileged to be invited.

- It is helpful to state at the outset that you have been allocated a certain amount of time to speak, and that you intend to allow some time for questions and discussion after your presentation is finished. You may want to invite people to interrupt you and ask questions as you go along, but that takes some doing! It is better for your peace of mind, at least in the early days of giving talks, to keep the questions to the end.

- Do not begin by 'running yourself down', or by apologising for your lack of experience. Of course, you may feel desperately nervous, but remember that you have been invited to give this talk and that you have already given it 'your best shot' in terms of preparation. Smile, and then get on with it. The audience will come to its own conclusions about what they think of you. Be proud that you are there and are going to do your best.

- Whether or not you have the use of a PA system, check at the outset whether you can be heard. If people ask you to speak louder, do so; but invite them to raise a hand if at any time they find you have reduced the volume.

- Remember the preparation you gave to the pace, clarity and delivery of your talk, and the 'music' of your voice. You will be surprised how easily all this goes out of your mind in the heat of the moment, and despite your best intentions you may begin to gabble. Remember to take pauses, to breathe deeply and to have short breaks in between sections. Take your cue from the audience: watch them, and that will give you a clear indication of whether you have their attention or not.

- Observe the golden rule of saying what you plan to say, say it and then stop. Do not try to improvise unless you are very experienced. Let the audience draw more out of you through their questions. This can be a bit daunting, but you can only do your best. You may become so absorbed in the discussion that you will find yourself answering questions easily, and in no time at all the meeting will be over. It is also helpful at the outset to give some pointers to what issues you are going to cover in the talk, and then at the very end to recap briefly before giving your final comments. This helps to clarify the structure of your talk in their minds, and acts as a useful 'aide memoire' for the audience.

- If you are using PowerPoint, avoid the temptation of turning to the screen behind you and talking to the slides. Keep talking to the audience; they can see the slides, and will prefer to see your face than the back of your head, especially if you are not using a PA system. Only turn to the screen if you need to point out something of key importance.

- If you are using videoclips that you are downloading from the Internet, check beforehand that it works successfully.

- If, during question time, you cannot answer a question, you may feel unnerved and begin to panic. Once again, the golden rule is to take your time; take a deep breath, and respond as honestly as you can. If there is nothing you can say, then it helps to reply by thanking the questioner for their comment and question, and simply saying that you are not sure but will find the answer and email it later. The audience will usually respond sympathetically to an honest reply. After all, it is better to be upfront and say you do not know, rather than prattle on inanely for five minutes, thereby demonstrating conclusively to them that what they suspected really is true.

- At the end, thank the audience for their attention and for their invitation. It is then often custom and practice for either the chair or a designated person to offer a vote of thanks to you. Enjoy the accolade and respond with a warm smile.
- If there is the facility or opportunity to obtain feedback from the audience, do make good use of it. If you have provided simple feedback sheets, invite people to complete them and leave them in the box at the door. (You did remember to put a box by the door beforehand, didn't you?) Or set up electronic feedback facilities and encourage people to use them.

## TACKLING THE GREMLINS

It would be wonderful to be able to say that each and every talk you give will be trouble-free, but that would be naively optimistic. Things can and do go wrong, and you will then have to think on your feet to decide how best to respond. Here are some classic examples of 'gremlins' at work:

- The PowerPoint suddenly freezes on you and refuses to respond to your urgent finger-tapping pleas.
- The internet site you are trying to access refuses to open.
- The bulb in the projector blows and there is no spare to replace it.
- In an unguarded moment, you knock your glass of water all over the table and your notes – it might even spill onto the chair's lap!
- There is an unexpected fire alarm.
- Someone's mobile phone goes off – or worse, your own mobile begins to play that dreadful tune you have been meaning to change for weeks.
- Someone in the front row falls asleep and begins to snore.
- People in the back row begin to chat among themselves.
- Someone arrives late and causes a great disturbance as they settle into their seat.
- The PA system screeches unexpectedly, or picks up conversations from the local taxi rank.
- Someone is taken ill during your talk.
- You drop your notes all over the floor.
- You experience an unexpected attack of hiccups or coughing, or your voice strength inexplicably fades.
- In the middle of the talk, you suddenly remember that you have not made arrangements for someone else to collect the children from school.
- You find the lack of personal hygiene with some people sitting near you almost overpowering.

- A spider, or a mouse, decides to run across the floor causing consternation to erupt.
- There is a power cut and you are all thrown into darkness.

In case you think these examples are from fantasyland, they have all been experienced in one form or another by the author, though thankfully not all on the same occasion.

Such gremlins will add an unwelcome piquancy to the occasion, and how you and others handle it will have to be decided upon there and then. One thing is clear: they will make the event doubly memorable! Sometimes a touch of humour will dispel the awkwardness, but use it with care and avoid inadvertently offending someone.

## Group exercise

With the help of your tutor or supervisor, respond to an invitation your group has received to give a talk to your local authority councillors about 'the highs and lows' of your professional training course, and any issues you need to bring to their attention.

## FINAL THOUGHTS

Giving talks can be some of the most enjoyable and rewarding occasions for you to use and develop your communication skills. But never forget the motto: To fail to prepare is to prepare to fail.

## REFERENCES AND FURTHER READING

Hopkins, G. (1998) *Plain English for Social Services: A Guide to Better Communication.* Lyme Regis: Russell House.
Thompson, N. (2011) *Effective Communication: A Guide for the People Professions,* 2nd edition. Basingstoke: Palgrave Macmillan.

### Web resources

There are several good websites available to help you develop your skills and confidence. For example:
Top Tips for Effective Presentations. Available at www.skillsyouneed.com/present/presentation-tips.html (accessed 25/11/19)

T

**RELATED CONCEPTS** non-verbal communication; overcoming fears and anxieties

**ENGAGING WITH THE PCF** context and organisations; knowledge; professionalism

**ENGAGING WITH THE NMC CODE** promote professionalism and trust

### Service user snippet

Jane (21), carer:

'I was asked to give a presentation to a large conference on my experiences as a carer. I wanted to do it but I was petrified – me? Speak to over 200 people? No way!! But a colleague took me through it and helped me plan carefully what I was going to say, and on the day everyone stood up and applauded me. They applauded ME!! I was so relieved and delighted it had gone so well.'

# TELEPHONE, SKYPING AND VIDEO CONFERENCING SKILLS

## TELEPHONE SKILLS

It is difficult to imagine any form of people-work taking place without the use of the telephone. It is a major means of communication between professionals, between agencies and between the professional worker and those with whom they are working. Given the explosion of mobile telephone provision, and its increasing sophistication, it may sound somewhat naive to suggest that people-workers need training in the professional use of this important communication tool. Surely we are all so confident with using telephones that we will adapt effortlessly to their professional usage?

The experience of student and trainee practitioners suggests otherwise. Many find themselves overawed by having to make a professional phone call; they dislike having to use the phone in front of other, more experienced colleagues in the office or on the ward; they can become 'tongue-tied', and they find it difficult to develop a professional approach. And yet a few simple guidelines are all that is needed to get people off to a good start.

---

## Activity

Spend some time ringing various organisations, firms, shops and service providers. Compare and contrast the ways in which these first impressions make an impact upon you. Was the welcoming message gabbled at speed, or were you able to take in what was being said? Was it pre-recorded or live? Did you have to select various options before you spoke to a real person? Did you find the message helpful or off-putting? Did their voice seem flat and monotonous, or did it come across in a warm, interesting way?

Now listen to your colleagues at work. How do they come across when they answer the phone? Is there an organisational expectation of the form of words to use when you answer the phone?

What can you learn from this exercise about how you will answer the phone at work when it rings? Write down what you think sounds best, and then try it out to see how it feels.

---

There are some obvious differences between face-to-face interviews and telephone conversations, and you need to develop the confidence to get the best out of each.

Your tone of voice can be very revealing: you can convey a lot of information through the careful development of the music of your own telephone voice. If you need any convincing of this, record yourself talking with someone sometime (with their permission) and then listen to the replay. You may be surprised that your voice is not as lively as you had thought. Or listen to the radio and appreciate the 'voice music' of words carefully delivered.

## Are you who you say you are?

You will tend to assume that the person ringing you for information is who they say they are, but can you be sure? If you know them well, it is not a problem, but in professional people-work you receive telephone enquiries all the time, and you have a professional responsibility to maintain confidentiality at all times. The Data Protection Act 2018 also lays a responsibility upon you to be extremely careful about what information you divulge about other people over the telephone.

Therefore, if you are not sure, ask for the name of the person who is ringing you, their location and the number for you to ring them back. This gives you time to check. Often, though, it is best to ask them to put their request in writing on official notepaper so that it can be dealt with properly.

Similarly, if you are the one making the call, explain who you are and why you require the information, and invite them to ring you back, giving your number and details. Before you ring, though, ask yourself whether this is information that you could reasonably expect to be given over the phone, or whether you should put the request in writing. How soon do you need this information? This could influence how you request it.

## Silence isn't always golden

In face-to-face interviews, you can often remain silent while the other person talks, because you can give encouragement to them with your facial expression, and some appropriate sounds of encouragement. On the telephone, it does not take much silence for it to become perplexing: the other person soon wonders if you are still there, or whether you have been cut off. This means that you need to be much more verbally active, simply to reassure the person that you are still there and are listening to them. This does not mean you have to use a lot more words – simply a more frequent use of 'mmm', 'yes', 'I see' and so on helps to oil the wheels of a non-visual conversation.

## An ear for detail

How often has an inexperienced worker put the phone down and realised too late that they have not taken down some vital piece of information, even as basic as the phone number and full name of the person they were speaking to. Remember the Activity? It is unlikely that you will have remembered the name of the person who was introducing themselves to you – the anxiety level of the first few seconds often blocks out these key details. It is very important, therefore, before the call is finished, that you ensure that key information is exchanged, and that you log it accordingly. After all, someone else may need to follow up this information and they will need the details about whom to ring.

### The dreaded answerphone

There is every chance that you will need to leave a message for someone, asking them to ring you back. Again, it is so easy not to give enough details – or to speak so quickly that the person at the other end does not stand a chance of taking down the information accurately. The golden rule is to keep it simple: speak slowly and clearly, say who you are, why you are ringing, give the day/date and time of your call, and the number for them to ring back. Depending on the circumstances, you may also wish to give a few brief details about what it is you wish to discuss with them. But do please remember that another person may pick up the message, thereby compromising confidentiality.

## MOBILE ETIQUETTE

The use of mobile phones as part of professional practice has increased enormously in recent years. There are distinct advantages to this. You can get in touch with your office when necessary, and they can update you quickly in emergencies. Your own personal safety is considerably enhanced if you have a mobile phone you can use. The more technically advanced mobiles also enable you to check your emails and 'surf the net' so that you can access information for immediate use in your meeting or with your service user or enquirer. And, of course, the use of text messaging opens up another new world of communication, although the temptation to use texting shorthand spellings should be avoided in formal written communications.

You should be particularly careful about sending personal information to a service user or patient by text messaging. Always check your agency guidelines and gain your manager's/supervisor's permission beforehand.

However, there are rules about mobile phone etiquette that are easy to overlook. You should turn them off during meetings and interviews in order to avoid disturbance and interruptions. If you are expecting an urgent call, set it to 'vibrate' and explain to the people you are with that you are expecting a call, and apologise in advance for any likely disturbance. It is unlawful to use the mobile phone while driving. And tempting though it may sometimes be, it is not professional to play games on your mobile while sitting at the back of a boring meeting.

One further point deserves consideration. You may find, from time to time, that a service user asks you for your mobile telephone number, or even your home telephone number or personal email address. Usually (but not always) this is because they value your help and support. But you are not their friend, and your personal life and space is separate from your professional life and space. If your agency is happy for you to give out your work mobile number, then you can give this out *if* you feel it is appropriate and boundaries are established about when they can or cannot ring you. But you should *never* disclose your personal information (or that of any other colleague). You will need to find your own form of words to use to explain this, but it is easiest simply to say: 'I'm sorry – I'm not allowed to give you that number/information – it's against the rules, and I would get into trouble.'

## Emojis and emoticons

There has been an explosion in the use and variety of emojis and emoticons, with text messages sometimes being littered with them. In personal communications these may well be a fun and often lighthearted way of enriching the text, with perhaps no harm done. In professional communications using text messages, however, there is good reason to think carefully about using them. Some workers may well feel that the use of emojis and emoticons softens and perhaps humanises their communication with a wide range of service users, especially young people who might thereby feel the worker was more 'on their wavelength'.

As a worker you always need to think carefully about the implications of the role you are fulfilling, and how professionally to communicate with people in your care. Emojis and emoticons may not always be as clear as you hope; they could be misunderstood; they might even cause offence. They might even undermine your professional relationship. The best advice is therefore to think twice before using them, and if in doubt leave them out.

---

### Group exercise

With the help of your tutor or supervisor, share together your experiences of using mobile text messages and emojis with your service users or patients. What are the advantages and potential pitfalls of using these forms of communication? Can you think of situations where their use might be helpful? Or situations where you definitely would not use them? Try a Google search to explore various ways in which emojis and emoticons are used to enhance contact with people with communication difficulties.

---

## SKYPING

The NHS is experimenting with the professional use of Skype for some GP consultations, and other agencies may well begin to explore this medium. The same issues and constraints apply as outlined above, but obviously you will have greater opportunity to engage visually. You need to be clear, however, about your agency guidelines for the use of Skype, and not allow this closer engagement to blur your professional relationships. The skills you need for successful Skyping are similar to those needed for video conferencing (see below).

# VIDEO CONFERENCING – HINTS AND TIPS

The advantages of video conferencing (VC) are self-evident. It can facilitate a wide cross-section of colleagues who need to meet and discuss issues of common concern or interest, without the need to travel long distances. VC can be a very effective use of time, and can enable decisions to be made more quickly in ways that involve all the key people concerned. It is also an important contribution to reducing the carbon footprint of face-to-face meetings.

But as with any interactive form of communication there can be challenges and difficulties that undermine the potential success of the interaction between those involved.

It may seem obvious, but the success or otherwise of a VC event will depend upon the reliability of the technology and the professionalism of everyone involved. If the equipment fails, or is not set up properly so that everyone can be clearly seen and heard, frustration levels will escalate. If the person chairing the VC conference is unable to operate with clear ground rules that give every participant the opportunity to contribute where appropriate, a lack of cohesion will quickly emerge. Careful planning and preparation is the key to a successful VC conference. Please also make sure you are familiar with the technology and what it can and cannot deliver. Some organisations, for example, have sophisticated systems with a 'mute microphone facility' to reduce the risk of feedback. And it is good practice to be able to contact the other participants by phone, email or text in case the technology lets you down in any way.

## Etiquette

All the basic ground rules for effective meetings also apply with video conferencing. Being and looking professional matters a lot (sorry – no sloppy T-shirts or inappropriate slogans on display even if you are working at home). Remember to introduce yourself clearly before you speak, especially if it is a large gathering. Anything that detracts from other people's concentration should be avoided – remember that everything you do will be seen by everyone else. It is easy to forget this, especially if geographically you are in different locations – the camera never lies!

Remember that those 'at the other end so to speak' will only see and hear what comes through the camera lens, so do avoid noisy settings, potential interruptions or excessive gesticulating. Remember to speak to the camera when it is your turn to contribute, and not to interrupt other speakers.

If you are chairing the VC, remember to thank people for their participation, and do ensure that everyone knows what has been agreed, how it will be recorded/minuted and who has responsibility for follow-up actions. Is a further VC needed? If so, plan the date and time together before you all sign off.

Finally, if for whatever reason the VC event did not go well, spend time afterwards identifying what needed to be done differently to ensure that next time it is more successful.

## Group exercise

With the help of your tutor or supervisor, set up a multi-agency VC event for your group. Divide into small groups, with each group taking on a role (e.g. arguing for or against the discharge of a vulnerable adult into inappropriate accommodation). Prepare your arguments and make the VC arrangements using whatever platform works best for you. Run the VC and evaluate the effectiveness of this form of communication. How might it have differed from, say, a telephone conference call?

## FINAL THOUGHTS

It is very easy to allow yourself to be controlled by the telephone, and to feel that you must be available to answer it 24/7. Emails, texts, social media messaging, diary reminders, can swamp your inbox – and that's not taking into account your personal and private stuff. Please try to remember that, in the end, the telephone is there to help you in your professional practice: as your servant, not as a controller. Ideally, you should have a separate phone for your work, but that isn't always possible. But even if you do have a separate one, do remember that there is no such thing as a phone that cannot be switched off. We know this is easy to say and difficult to do, but there is life outside of work!

## REFERENCES AND FURTHER READING

Allen, G. and Langford, D. (2007) *Effective Interviewing in Social Work and Social Care*. Basingstoke: Palgrave Macmillan.

Koprowska, J. (2019) *Communication and Interpersonal Skills in Social Work*, 5th edition. Exeter: Learning Matters.

Trevithick, P. (2012) *Social Work Skills and Knowledge: A Practice Handbook*, 3rd edition. Maidenhead: Open University Press.

**RELATED CONCEPTS** chairing meetings; establishing a professional relationship; information and communication technology (ICT); reflective practice

**ENGAGING WITH THE PCF** context and organisations; skills and interventions; professionalism

**ENGAGING WITH THE NMC CODE** practise effectively; promote professionalism and trust

T

## Service user snippets

Vibhuti (28), social work student:

'On my first placement I was in an open-plan office with six other people and I was the only student. Every time I had to make a phone call I was so nervous about being overheard. I thought people would put me down and it began to get to me – I dreaded it ringing! Fortunately my supervisor realised what I was going through, and suggested that I spent a week in her office making and receiving phone calls – that boosted my confidence because she gave me helpful feedback, and after that I was fine.'

Darren (19), social work student:

'I was so proud of myself on placement for setting up a video conferencing meeting with various professionals up and down the country. But the signal failed and I had left all the contact details for everyone back in my office. I was so embarrassed! But people came to my rescue and eventually it worked a treat. But never discount gremlins!'

# TIME MANAGEMENT

How you manage your time professionally communicates important messages to others about how you view them and the work you undertake with them. In western society at least, great store is put on punctuality: to arrive half an hour late is tantamount to insulting the person(s) waiting for you. It conveys in terms of non-verbal communication the message that they are not important enough for you to put yourself out for them and to be on time.

And yet we all know how difficult this can be at times. You may set out with every good intention of being on time for all your appointments, but people-work is a complex activity, full of the unexpected. It only takes a sudden crisis for your schedule to be thrown into chaos. And you can become very resentful when the people you have kept waiting are angry at you for letting them down and are not willing to accept what (to you) are compelling reasons for lateness.

There are no absolutely foolproof strategies for perfect time management, and certainly in the early days of your people-work career you will at times struggle to balance the many, sometimes conflicting, demands upon your time. If only there was an easy way to learn how to prioritise!

---

## Activity

Look back over your diary/electronic calendar for the past two weeks. How well do you feel you managed and planned your time? Were there any occasions when you were unavoidably delayed? How did you handle this? How might you deal with it differently?

---

Good time management comes with experience, and it is a skill we all have to develop for ourselves. There are some useful tips that will help. These include:

- Keep your appointments diary/electronic calendar in some detail. For example, note the address and telephone number (if available) of people, meetings and visits you arrange so that they are easily to hand if you need to contact them while out of the office. A quick telephone call to say you have been delayed will help to defuse people's anxieties about why you are late, and will reassure them that you have not forgotten them.
- Allow time for travelling and breaks. If you are not sure of an area, allow enough time for getting a bit lost on the first time you go there. Not everyone has 'sat-nav' facilities, and even the joys of Google Maps or similar electronic direction finders cannot guarantee total success against road works, accidents and rush-hour jams. If you are planning on several visits in one day, allow time 'for you' in

your schedule, for refreshments, comfort breaks and unwinding, and for making notes on each visit afterwards so that they do not all blur into one. Try not to allow yourself to be run ragged by giving yourself too ambitious a list to tackle in any one day. If your agency provides you with a laptop, you will be able to record each visit there and then, but not everyone yet has this facility provided for them.

- When you arrange home visits, think about what else you have to do that day, and in your appointment letter, or when you speak face to face, give the time you hope to arrive, and say that you will make every effort to be punctual, but explain that there may be occasions where something unavoidable crops up and you may be delayed. Forewarned is forearmed.

- Know what are your best times and your worst times. If you are a morning person, for example, you will probably want to ensure that you tackle the most demanding of tasks when your energy levels are at their best, and leave the more mundane things for later in the day when you can be a bit more on 'autopilot'.

- Ensure that you put regular events into the diary well in advance. Team meetings and supervision sessions are good examples of this, but it is also helpful to allocate some time each week to catching up with reading, filing and record keeping.

- Think about your annual leave entitlement and how you want to take it. Do you have free rein, or is there an agency culture about when leave can be taken? Plan ahead so that you have the breaks you need and deserve to avoid burn out.

- Ensure that really important events, like attendance at court, case conferences and key meetings, are put into your diary as soon as you know of them.

- If you keep a social diary as well as a work-based diary, you need to be doubly vigilant. If you fail to take into account an important birthday, anniversary or social function, and plan to work late that evening, you will find your popularity ratings plummeting with certain people close to you. For this reason, many people keep a basic note of personal matters in their work diary to avoid such clashes. Again, to miss these events when you could reasonably have planned not to, is to communicate something about your priorities to the other person(s) involved. And there is life outside work – or there ought to be – to keep you lively and vibrant as a person. Electronic diaries, of course, present added complications if others can make appointments on your behalf. It is important, therefore, to ensure that you keep control by making it clear when you are, and are not, available.

## A NOTE OF CAUTION

Diaries contain information both about you and those with whom you are working and visiting. You need to take reasonable steps to ensure that confidentiality is maintained in your diary. But most of all you need to keep it very safe. A lost diary is a multi-dimensional disaster to be avoided at all costs. So do keep it secure, and don't leave it unattended in the car or anywhere else.

## A USEFUL TIP

If you use a paper-based diary, it is a good idea to photocopy your diary every now and then so that a spare copy of your appointments is available in the event of your diary going missing for some reason. In moments of stress, we can all do things we regret, and a mislaid diary can cause all manner of complications. A photocopy kept in a safe place really can save the day. Alternatively, it may be useful to save such information electronically, for example on a smartphone, laptop or in your Outlook calendar.

## FINAL THOUGHTS

Although time is a very measured, and measurable, phenomenon, it is also a social and an emotional construct. To be late in some cultures is almost to insult people, whereas in other settings the concept of being 'late' hardly seems to occur to people. In our own lives, time can drag, stand still or fly by. And, of course, for some professional people, time is money. Time therefore is a multi-layered phenomenon, and in our professional lives we need to be aware of its many complexities, as well as ensuring that we make the best use of it in our work.

## REFERENCES AND FURTHER READING

Stogden, C. and Kitely, R. (2010) *Study Skills for Social Workers*. London: Sage.
Thompson, N. (2006) *Promoting Workplace Learning*. Bristol: Policy Press.
Thompson, N. (2015) *People Skills*, 4th edition. Basingstoke: Palgrave Macmillan.

**RELATED CONCEPTS** endings; establishing a professional relationship; reflective practice

**ENGAGING WITH THE PCF** context and organisations; professionalism

**ENGAGING WITH THE NMC CODE** practise effectively; promote professionalism and trust

### Service user snippet

Johann (36), social worker:

'I can't tell you how mortified I was to have lost my work diary. One minute I had it but then … I must have put it down somewhere in a stressful moment … it had so much information in it as well – it was as if I had lost an arm or a leg … I felt totally disempowered, as well as guilty having to tell my manager. I was given a verbal warning, and rightly so. I'll never allow that to happen again … ever.'

# TRICKY TOPICS: SEXUALITY AND DEATH

Experienced and inexperienced workers alike may respond in a similar way to this topic: *tell me any topic that isn't tricky!* And of course they are right. People-work in all its many guises is challenging and we have to think on our feet – quickly! Reflexive practice recognises this, and reminds us that as soon as we go into 'automatic mode' in our dealings with others we have begun to lose the plot; or – more importantly – we have begun to lose that essential humanity which characterises all good people-work.

There is also the danger that by labelling something – or someone – as tricky, or difficult, we are putting them into a box labelled 'potentially unhelpable'. What we should be asking, however, is what is it about us and our values and attitudes that makes us feel that 'these people' (there we go again!) are tricky customers, or that somehow we don't feel adequate when working with them?

Having said that, there are some situations which are particularly demanding: breaking bad news, exploring issues around religion and spirituality, whistleblowing, dealing with 'wrong' messages and everything surrounding abusive relationships all fall into this category and are explored in various ways in this book.

Two other themes, however, deserve particular attention: sexuality and death. Not least because such topics deeply affect all of us, who we are and what we believe. Our own values, attitudes and prejudices are never far from the surface, and will impact upon how we relate to other people. So the initial focus with such topics needs to be not on other people but upon us. The importance of self-awareness is a crucial component in any people-worker's armoury.

---

## Activity

Spend a few moments thinking about each of these questions:

- What are the issues, questions and puzzlements that spring to mind when you think about sexuality and death?
- How do you understand your own sexuality?
- What do think or believe about death?

---

## SEXUALITY

When reflecting on your own sexuality, did you find yourself thinking in rigid categories, such as 'male or female', 'gay or straight', or did you sense that the picture is much more complex, richer even, than that? Did you reflect on bisexual or transgender implications for our understanding of our sexuality? We are beginning to realise that there is a fluidity in everyone's sexuality that enriches our understanding and appreciation of diversity.

Having said that, there are many people for whom such fluidity is a worrying threat, or challenge even, to their deeply held moral or religious views. You may include yourself in this, and therefore find it very difficult to accept the value base of people-work that celebrates diversity in this aspect of life.

Wherever you are on this spectrum of views, the important point to stress is self-awareness so that you do not allow your own views or prejudices to get in the way of the work you will be doing with people whose lifestyle may differ radically from your own.

---

### Group exercise

With the help of your tutor or supervisor, explore together some of the implications for professional practice arising from our developing awareness of LGBTQ+ issues. There is a developing richness in the language and understanding of these issues. Do you fully appreciate what LGBTQ+ represents? Visit www.stonewall.org.uk or https://ok2bme.ca/ (a Canadian resource) to help you develop your awareness and understanding. Identify some specific issues for your own professional practice and how these might be addressed.

---

Sexual abuse

There is, however, one further issue that may deeply perplex or upset you: sexual abuse. To work with people who have committed sexual abuse, especially with vulnerable children, makes significant demands upon workers, both professionally and emotionally. To witness the impact of abuse upon innocent victims can at times be gut-wrenching. Operation Yewtree, which investigated the abusive behaviour of Jimmy Saville in 2012, is but one of many disturbing examples of the challenge of abusive behaviour and the need to protect vulnerable young people and children. To work with perpetrators of abuse is never easy, and should never be undertaken by inexperienced or underqualified practitioners. Nevertheless, even at an early stage in your career, whether in social work, nursing or social care, you may well encounter both victims and perpetrators, and therefore you need to think through your personal and professional response and approach. The importance of good supervision, a well-prepared plan of action and the opportunity to reflect upon the impact such work is having on you, cannot be over-emphasised.

**T**

## DEATH AND DYING

As with sexuality, so too death raises profound issues. Whether or not you have experienced the death and loss of someone close to you, there is an inevitability to it which makes everyone pause to reflect. For those with a specific religious faith, death may be understood as being more of a threshold to a future spiritual existence than a literal 'dead end' to life. Death also comes with particularly jagged edges, especially with the death of children; the ravages of war, disaster or disease; life-limiting conditions; suicide, murder or serious accidents. The list seems endless but the impact remains similar: lives are torn apart, families are decimated, hopes and dreams are destroyed. The big questions (*Why do such things happen? What is our place in the universe? Can we make sense of what has happened?*) all churn around inside us.

If you find yourself caught up in a caring capacity with someone who has experienced these emotional upheavals, you will inevitably wonder how best to respond. What is safe to assume is that a 'good listening to' will always be appreciated, and that imposing our own views, opinions and beliefs, however well intentioned, will seldom be appreciated. In such situations, not knowing the answers (always supposing that there are some!) is common ground, not least because the world view that we may have chosen may not resonate with the other person's beliefs. Active listening skills can enable you to make an empathic response to someone going through emotional and spiritual turmoil. But ultimately we are faced with mystery, and however uncomfortable that may be, we do ourselves and those whom we seek to help a great disservice if we pretend otherwise.

## FINAL THOUGHTS

This very brief introduction to two tricky topics is intended to get you thinking and reflecting, and wanting to learn more. Spend some time choosing a book or visit a relevant website on these themes to study the issues more deeply, in order to enrich and deepen your knowledge and self-awareness.

 ## REFERENCES AND FURTHER READING

Cowburn, M. (2016) *Social Work with Sex Offenders* (Social Work in Practice series). Bristol: Policy Press.

Hicks, S. (2015) 'Social work and gender: an argument for practical accounts', *Qualitative Social Work*, 14 (4): 471–87.

Holloway, M. and Moss, B. (2010) *Spirituality and Social Work*. Basingstoke: Palgrave Macmillan.

Thompson, N. (2012) *Grief and its Challenges*. Basingstoke: Palgrave Macmillan.

Thompson, N. (2016) *Anti-Discriminatory Practice*, 6th edition. Basingstoke: Palgrave Macmillan.

**RELATED CONCEPTS** acceptance; active listening; breaking bad news; emotional intelligence (EI); empathy; loss; religion; spirituality

**ENGAGING WITH THE PCF** critical reflection; knowledge; values and ethics

**ENGAGING WITH THE NMC CODE** prioritise people; promote professionalism and trust

---

### Service user snippets

Barry (23), physically disabled service user:

> 'I knew as soon as I started talking to my social worker about being transgender that he strongly disapproved … I just froze and couldn't speak.'

Siobhan (25), single parent:

> 'It was such a relief when my support worker took my religious views as a Muslim seriously. I could have cried with relief.'

# WHISTLEBLOWING

'Whistleblowing' is the term used when a worker reports malpractice or wrong doing at work. This is known formally as 'making a disclosure in the public interest'. Inevitably, the communication skills required are of the highest order for this to be done effectively.

To be in this position is perhaps one of the most difficult and, at times, lonely and potentially isolating experiences you can have. The temptation to keep quiet and to hope that the problem will go away can be immense; the decision to challenge and/ or report your concerns can sometimes require great courage, as evidenced in the Mid Staffordshire NHS Hospital Trust scandal (Francis, 2013).

## Activity

Spend a few moments compiling a list of poor practice that you feel would justify your becoming a whistleblower. How do you think that this action would be received by your management, your colleagues and the person whom you are reporting? Do you feel you would be supported? Would you feel anxious or frightened in any way about whatever consequences might flow from your actions? Make a note of these and refer to them as this discussion unfolds.

If you have completed this Activity thoughtfully, you will have already realised how complex and potentially 'scary' this situation can be. Perhaps, too, you will have realised that whistleblowing is a tactic of the last resort: crucially important, but nonetheless not to be considered as the first step to take.

If you find yourself in this sort of situation – let's say, by way of illustration, that a colleague is misappropriating agency funds, or acting abusively towards a service user, or you discover that patients in your hospital are being ill-treated, neglected or put at serious risk – you need to think carefully about what to do. The following checklist will help you clarify your thinking:

1   Are you certain about this? Is it merely a suspicion, or do you have hard evidence? If you are going to make an allegation about a colleague, you must be very sure of your facts. Imagine how you would feel if someone 'got hold of the wrong end of the stick' and accused you unfairly of a misdemeanour.
2   Check your agency policy to see, first of all, whether there is a whistleblowing policy. More and more agencies are required to have one, and various training and education course providers are required to have one in place so that students and workers are clear about such matters.

- If you do have a policy, read it through carefully: it should give you a step-by-step procedure to follow. It should also reassure you that it is illegal for you to be victimised in any way as a result of your report, irrespective of the eventual outcome. Things may be uncomfortable for a while, but you should not be in any way penalised.

- If you cannot find a policy, ask someone to help you locate it. This may feel difficult, of course, as people will immediately begin to wonder why you are asking. You will have to decide how to approach this. Sometimes you can explain that you are doing a comparative study or research project on whistleblowing as part of a course you are on, or out of general interest. It is always a good idea to look at other agencies' policies anyway. If you draw a blank, especially if you feel uncomfortable about probing further, then seek advice. To whom you turn will depend very much upon your status within the agency. If you are a student, for example, you should always talk first to your supervisor or practice educator and/or your academic tutor. If, however, you are a worker in the agency, you may feel it will help to talk to an independent body for advice and information such as Citizens Advice. This process of fact-finding is important as it will help you decide the best course of action.

3   Find an ally whom you can trust, with whom you can discuss things confidentially and seek support. This can be a very worrying and stressful situation to be in, and having a good supporter can sometimes make all the difference if the going gets tough.

4   Decide whether you can approach the person directly in some way. This is not easy, but it is worth considering at the outset. If you can find a quiet moment, you could tell the other person that you hope you are wrong, but that you have noticed what seems to be going on, and that this will put you in a difficult position if it continues. It is probably not wise to enter into a detailed discussion, but it will be instructive to hear the response that your statement elicits. If it is true, the other person will have been warned, and will have to do something to put the situation right.

5   If this course of action is not possible for whatever reason, then the time has come to talk to someone in authority – your supervisor or immediate line manager, and perhaps your union representative. They should be able to advise you about what to do next. They may tell you that they will take the responsibility to follow up your concerns and allegations without bringing your name into it, and to see that matters are properly dealt with. Unless there are compelling reasons to doubt what is being said to you, you should let the manager take it forward, and try to let the matter rest at that point. But do make a note of what you have done and said for your own records, and keep it in a safe place.

6   If all else fails, then you need to activate the formal whistleblowing procedure by writing to the senior manager or Chief Executive Officer (CEO), outlining your concerns and allegations and citing relevant evidence in support of them. Mark the letter 'Strictly private and confidential' and keep a copy for your own records. Do not send it electronically – it is not always possible to guarantee that it will remain confidential or be seen only by the person to whom you

have sent it. If the CEO needs to copy it to key people, that will be his or her responsibility.

7   How the agency deals with this may vary. Best practice suggests that you should be called to a meeting to discuss your allegations with the CEO in confidence, but sometimes all you may receive is a brief letter of acknowledgement. Occasionally, you may not even receive that, and you may be left wondering what is happening. You will have discharged your responsibility by sending it, but you may also wish to follow it up by asking whether the matter has been resolved.

8   Always bear in mind that the best agencies will welcome whistleblowing and will want to make the process as straightforward as possible in order to maintain their reputation for high standards. Indeed, anything which undermines that, or goes against the grain of the agency's value base, deserves to be challenged, and should be welcomed. The agency should have the self-same set of concerns and value base that caused you to be concerned in the first place.

---

## Group exercise

With the help of your tutor or supervisor, identify some examples of whistleblowing in your organisation. What were the issues? What was the outcome? How well do you think the issue was handled? Do you feel confident that you could 'blow the whistle' if the need arose?

---

## FINAL THOUGHTS

However much you may agree in your head with what has been said about whistleblowing, when it becomes real for you, your heart and 'gut' may well tell another story. You may find, for example, that the aftershock may be more painful for you than you had expected; you may be made to feel very uncomfortable, victimised even. If this happens, always keep a careful note of what is happening, and if necessary lodge a complaint or a grievance. Seek legal advice; approach human resources/personnel staff/your union representative to help you clarify the situation. As a last resort, look for another job which better reflects your own values. This is not necessarily going to be easy, but matters of deep principle and conscience are of such importance that you will know deep down that you have to do what is right if you are going to be able to continue living with yourself. It will be this sense of doing what you know to be right that will sustain you in darker times.

 ## REFERENCES AND FURTHER READING

Alford, C.F. (2002) *Broken Lives and Organisational Power*. New York: Cornell University Press.

**W**

Bowers, J., Lewis, J., Fodder, M. and Mitchell, J. (2017) *Whistleblowing: Law and Practice*, 3rd edition. Oxford: Oxford University Press.

Francis, R. (2013) *Report of the Mid Staffordshire NHS Foundation Trust Public Inquiry*. Norwich: TSO.

Kohn, S. (2011) *Whistleblower's Handbook – A Step-by-Step Guide to Doing What's Right and Protecting Yourself*. Guilford, CT: Lyons Press.

Parker, J. (2010) *Effective Practice Learning in Social Work*, 2nd edition. Exeter: Learning Matters.

n.b. Whistleblowing law is located in the Employment Rights Act (1996) as amended by the Public Interest Disclosure Act (1998).

## Web resources

Citizens Advice – www.citizensadvice.org.uk (accessed 11/09/2019)
Public Concern at Work, the whistleblowing charity – www.pcaw.co.uk (accessed 11/09/2019)

**RELATED CONCEPTS** establishing a professional relationship; overcoming fears and anxieties; reflective practice; supervision

**ENGAGING WITH THE PCF** critical reflection and analysis; contexts and organisations; professional leadership; professionalism; values and ethics

**ENGAGING WITH THE NMC CODE** preserve safety; promote professionalism and trust

### Service user snippet

Kelly (28), nurse:

'I can honestly say that when I decided to report a colleague's malpractice to my manager I was terrified I would be made to suffer. But to my delight I was taken seriously and steps were taken to improve the team's overall performance and values. But I know of other colleagues elsewhere whose lives were made a misery when they blew the whistle. We need more protection if we are going to improve our service.'

# WRONG MESSAGES

The discussion about non-verbal communication skills emphasises how important it is to be aware of 'wrong' messages we can convey to people sometimes without being aware of it. Turning up late to see people can give them the impression, for example, that they are not very important and that we do not care very much about them. More serious, however, is the possibility of giving wrong messages to the people with whom we work. This is often about workers not maintaining appropriate professional boundaries in their relationships with people.

For example, being friendly towards those with whom we work is an important aspect of establishing a professional relationship, within which we can do some important work with people. It is an aspect of empathy. But we are not actually becoming friends with the other person. Our relationship is established for a specific purpose; once accomplished, the relationship comes to an end – or, as we say, *job done*. It would be wholly inappropriate to keep in touch with the person, or to have coffee with them or go on a day out with them, because this would take the relationship into a more personal rather than professional sphere.

It has to be admitted that this boundary is not always easy to maintain. In some aspects of people-work it is often helpful to meet the person on what may be called 'neutral territory' – in other words, not at your office or in their home. Work with disadvantaged young people or a young carer, for example, may sometimes be far more effective if the worker sees them in town, in a coffee bar or internet café. It conveys an important message about meeting people in territory that they feel comfortable in. But the relationship must still remain professional.

Difficulties arise because, as human beings, we have feelings, and sometimes deep attraction to each other. A person who has been going through emotional turmoil may feel hugely grateful to you for your time, concern, and your friendly, caring approach. They may feel that you have made all the difference to their life, and a deep sense of gratitude can begin to form. They may want to show this gratitude through physical affection to you. And because feelings can be two-way, you may also begin to experience strong feelings for the other person, stemming first from a sense of protection perhaps, or from wanting them to recover from whatever is afflicting them; but this can then move on towards a feeling of physical attraction. The service user may feel they are falling in love with you: their feelings may be reciprocated, and a sexual relationship may then follow (see the entry on transference on pp. 132–134).

## Activity

Think carefully about some of the work you have undertaken with people where you felt a degree of physical attraction towards them. How did you handle this? Are there some situations in which you feel personally that you would be more vulnerable than others? How will you plan to deal with such scenarios?

It must be said categorically that this is both unprofessional and unacceptable behaviour that flouts professional codes of conduct. Cases of this nature almost always result in disciplinary proceedings being taken against the worker, who will be deemed to have breached their position of trust, and to have exploited someone who was deemed vulnerable.

But we live in the real world of flesh, blood and lust, and it would be naive to pretend that in your professional relationships you do not, from time to time, find someone you are working with extremely attractive physically. It is important, therefore, that you take steps not only to protect yourself against any accusation of inappropriate conduct, but also to guard against entering into physical and sexual relationships. Partnership working does not mean you can become partners!

In guarding against the over-stepping of boundaries with service users, there are several important points to bear in mind:

- Always ensure that the place and time where you meet is appropriate.
- If need be, ensure that you are not working alone with the other person.
- If feelings of attraction to a service user begin to occur, raise the issue with your practice educator, supervisor or manager at an early stage so that you can discuss how best to deal with it.
- Be reflective: what are these feelings within you telling you about yourself, your level of self-awareness, your need to be loved and to be seen to be attractive, and your own personal relationships?
- Ensure that the non-verbal communications between you and the other person are kept within the boundaries of the professional relationship. Do not underestimate the impact of a warm look, a deep smile or a physical touch: to someone who is feeling unloved, vulnerable and uncared for, it may be easy to misunderstand what is being communicated.
- If you sense that the other person is becoming too interested in you 'as you', remind them of the professional nature of the relationship, and always end the interview in a low-key, businesslike manner. You may even wish to use their formal title rather than their first name when saying goodbye, just to reinforce this message.

There are some other strategies that some people-workers choose to adopt, such as the wearing of a ring on their wedding finger, irrespective of whether they are in a committed relationship. Some workers – both male and female – feel that this is an important reinforcement of their professional boundaries. There will, of course, be others who fiercely eschew such a practice as being wholly dishonest, regarding it as a 'game' that they do not wish to play. This is for you to decide.

> ## Group exercise
>
> With the help of your tutor or supervisor, discuss relevant strategies for dealing with the issues raised in this chapter. Have there been any examples in your own organisation where these issues have gone badly wrong? What can you learn from this for your own practice?

## FINAL THOUGHTS

It is important to reinforce the principal issue in all of this: we enter into professional relationships with people for a distinct and clearly negotiated purpose, which has an end in sight. Best practice will never lose sight of the endings from the very beginning, and will always seek to be evaluating and assessing the progress being made towards achieving agreed objectives. The quality of the empathic professional relationship that we establish will be crucial to achieving these objectives, but once that relationship becomes an end in itself, we will have crossed a vital boundary.

## REFERENCES AND FURTHER READING

Beckett, C., Maynard, A. and Jordan, P. (2017) *Values and Ethics in Social Work*, 3rd edition. London: Sage.

Cooper, F. (2012) *Professional Boundaries in Social Work and Social Care: A Practical Guide to Understanding, Maintaining and Managing Your Professional Boundaries*. London: Jessica Kingsley.

Ruch, G. Turney, D. and Ward. A, (2018) *Relationship-Based Social Work, Getting to the Heart of Practice*, 2nd Edition. London: Jessica Kingsley.

Rutter, L. and Brown, K. (2019) Critical *Thinking and Professional Judgement for Social Work (Post-Qualifying Social Work Practice Series)*, 5th edition. London: Sage.

 Web resources

Social Work England – www.socialworkengland.org.uk (accessed 11/09/19)

**RELATED CONCEPTS** barrier gestures; endings; establishing a professional relationship; non-verbal communication; supervision

**ENGAGING WITH THE PCF** critical reflection and analysis; empathy; professionalism; values and ethics

**ENGAGING WITH THE NMC CODE** practise effectively; promote professionalism and trust

## Service user snippet

Corinne (46), support worker:

'I had no idea why my service user seemed so "off" with me. I know I was late yet again but with my caseload that is hardly surprising and the last thing I need is ear-ache from someone who doesn't understand the pressures I work under. But then she told me how my persistent lateness made her feel undervalued and as if I didn't care about her. It was a light-bulb moment for me – I had no idea she felt that way.'

# INDEX